THE LD
CHRONICLES

THE LD CHRONICLES

A STORY ABOUT A PHYSICIAN AND HIS MISSING PROSTATE

BRAD RANDALL, MD

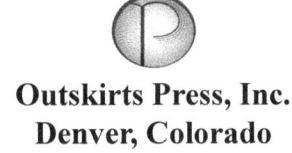

Outskirts Press, Inc.
Denver, Colorado

Outskirts Press, Inc.
http://www.outskirtspress.com

ISBN: 978-1-4327-7030-3

Library of Congress Control Number: 2011924066

Outskirts Press and the "OP" logo are trademarks belonging to Outskirts Press, Inc.

PRINTED IN THE UNITED STATES OF AMERICA

Dedicated to my – and all – Dear Sainted Wives

Contents

Disclaimer

In the beginning, as I began to consider the consequences of documenting how cancer forced a man to separate himself from his prostate, I began to wonder: Exactly what right do I have to write about what, in the greater scheme of things, is a relatively trivial matter? I mean, in the greater scope of things, this usually isn't life or death stuff.

Clearly, we know that there are thousands of people who have faced down terrible cancers, endured horrible surgeries, suffered through physical and sprit sapping chemotherapies, only to be ultimately forced to accept that these Herculean efforts were all in vain. Everyday we watch war veterans coming home with horrific injuries – traumatic brain injuries, loss of limbs, battlefield nightmares – all tales of sacrifice and courage. The world is full of stories of people grappling, some successfully and some not, with horrific physical and mental challenges.

How can I even presume that a story about a misplaced prostate could be presented without first hearing from those who have truly suffered and battled with the worst that life could throw at them? The answer, as I thought more about the question, was essentially that I couldn't make such a presumption, which left me to mentally shit-can the project, and that was that.

But the idea of a prostate-less story kept going through my mind, most often during that time of the day – my morning constitutional and shower – that I usually reserve for thinking deep thoughts. Eventually it came to me that my justification for writing this little epistle wasn't because it was a tale of overcoming horrible and unusual obstacles it was, in fact, just the opposite.

I truly want to hear those stories of how someone overcame, or ultimately didn't overcome, a great challenge in their life. But in reality, I know that these great stories gain much of their power from the fact that they are about things that one can reasonably expect won't happen to the reader or their loved ones.

I believe that my story deserves a hearing not because it is so unique and gripping, but rather because it is so common. Physicians believe that were we to look carefully at every elderly man's prostate, we would find cancer. Fortunately we don't look all that carefully -- yet about one in six men will have a diagnosis of prostate cancer during their life. Somewhere around 200,000 men a year will have prostate cancer surgery or radiation therapy.

While you may never know a veteran who struggles to walk again with a prosthetic leg (and we all deserve to hear his or her story), the odds are overwhelming that you, or someone you know and love, will have to deal with prostate cancer and its therapies.

I make no pretense that my story is, or is not, in any way average or usual. I have no way of knowing what "average" is, and seriously doubt that there is any "average" or "usual" story to tell. I have reviewed the prostate cancer literature, but perhaps less scientifically and more meaningfully, I have talked with many men who have preceded and followed me along this path. Some have had more problems, some fewer, than I encountered. But I believe that what follows will be informative, and hopefully helpful, to those men and their families who, as I did, find themselves looking at coping with prostate cancer.

When I was contemplating my prostatectomy I actively sought out men I knew who had had the procedure, in order to seek their advice. I wanted to hear, "first hand," what I might expect. I write this story of my adventure to offer both to those who are facing a prostatectomy, but perhaps equally importantly, to their partners who might not have a prostate-free male friend to ask, a "first hand" account.

I have tried to paint this story as humorously as possible. If, at times, it goes a little over the top, please accept my apologies, if for no other reason than I'm an incurable punner. For those of you who don't happen to know a forensic pathologist, gallows humor often is part of our work, and can be a great aid in dealing with things that otherwise would make you cry.

{Author's note: What follows is a combination of "my story" and a little didactic teaching about anatomy, medicine, and prostate physiology. I believe that both are important elements for any potential reader. But I also think it is helpful to separate the two threads. I therefore have italicized the teaching segments, which I hope will make it a little more helpful to find and reference the "medical" versus personal parts of the story.}

A Glossary of Terms

Before I begin, there are some terms and words that might need defining and explaining, which aren't necessarily the same things. Some of the words and terms below may truly need defining, and I hope what is provided is helpful. But mostly they are words and terms that are well-known to most everyone, but whose use posed a potential problem in the text. For several words and terms, I had to decide exactly which of their many synonyms to use. The definitions provide a way to work through the tension between those words your doctor might use and the alternative definitions that you might use at home or in the locker room.

Where possible I have followed each word or term with the definition given in *Dorland's Medical Dictionary* and the battered *Webster's* dictionary on my shelf. I realize that for many of these words I don't even begin to plumb the depths of the potential other equivalent words more commonly used in day-to-day speech. If I have left out your favorite synonym, I apologize. Please chalk it up to an attempt to avoid overtly grossing anyone out, a desire to keep this section relatively short, and perhaps an inadequate knowledge of the pornographic literature and an insular upbringing.

For those that might find themselves offended by the time you have reached the end of the list, perhaps you should stop reading. This is a story about intimate things that you wouldn't discuss in "polite" company. There probably are even some things which many would feel uncomfortable discussing in "impolite" company. I have no desire to be lascivious with any of this. These words, and my story, are about human sexuality and those other things human males do with their penises (see definition below).

Sexual intercourse/Sex:

Webster's: 1. "A sexual connection esp. between humans."
Coitus – "The natural conveying of semen to the female reproductive tract."
Copulate – "To engage in sexual intercourse."
Dorland's: see Coitus,
Coitus – "Sexual union between individuals of the opposite sex."
Copulate – "Sexual congress."

All I can say is that if you were an alien from Mars and read those definitions, you wouldn't have any idea what humans are doing for fun or where babies of most animals come from. Why don't they just say, "The insertion of a penis into a vagina or some other bodily orifice for sexual pleasure or reproduction."

On the street synonyms vary from making love to screwing, fucking, doing the deed, banging, and if I read a different type of literature more often, undoubtedly the list would go on and on. For the purpose of this book I think I will stick with "having sex."

Penis:

Webster's: "A male organ of copulation."

Dorland's: "The male organ of copulation, [but wait, it goes on] comprising a root, body, and extremity, or glans penis. The root is attached to the descending portions of the pubic bone by the cura, the latter being the extremities of the corpora cavernosa. The body consists of two parallel cylindrical bodies, the _corpora cavernosa_, and beneath them the corpus _spongiosum_, through which the urethra passes. The glans is covered with mucous membrane and ensheathed by the prepuce, or foreskin."

On the street the list of synonyms must be huge. In part the list would include at least dick, cock, member, johnson, jones, little Willy, and prick. I suspect that I, like many other men and their partners, often choose to label their penises with their own pet names. I share a great deal in this book, but that particular name is private.

Which leads me to the problem of what to call this most intimate, private, and so very important part of my body? "Penis" seems just too clinical and impersonal. The street names seem to strip it of its dignity. As you will read, my urologist, once in need of examining my penis, said without hesitation, "Okay, let's take a look at your 'little buddy.'" That seemed somehow appropriate at the time, and it's what I think I'll stick with. My penis henceforth shall be called "My Little Buddy."

Erection:

Webster's: a. "The state marked by firm turgid form and erect position of a previously flaccid bodily part containing cavernous tissue when that tissue becomes dilated with blood." b. "An occurrence of such a state in the penis or clitoris." What would have been nice to have added to the definition, "A requisite for sexual intercourse."

Dorland's: "The condition of being made rigid and elevated." (And this is a medical dictionary?)

On the street: Most commonly hard-on or woody with undoubtedly many more that I haven't heard. I will stick with erection.

Ejaculate/Semen:

Webster's (n. ejaculate): *"The semen released by an ejaculation."*
Semen – *"A viscid whitish fluid of the male reproductive tract consisting of spermatozoa suspended in secretions of accessory glands."*

Dorland's (n. ejaculate/ejaculum): *"The fluid discharged at ejaculation in the male, consisting of the secretions of Cowper's gland, epididymis, ductus deferens, seminal vesicles, and prostate, and containing the spermatozoa."*
Semen – "See ejaculum above."

On the street commonly referred to as cum, jisim, spunk, or seed. I personally like "ejaculate," but I suppose "semen" is more commonly used and I'll use them interchangeably.

Impotence/impotent:

Webster's: *"Unable to copulate."*

Dorland's: *"Lack of power: chiefly of copulative power or virility. It may be atonic, due to paralysis of the motor nerves (nervi erigentes) without evidence of lesion of the central nervous system; paretic, due to lesion in the central nervous system, particularly in the spinal cord; psychic, dependent on mental complex; symptomatic, due to some other disorder, such as injury to nerves in the perineal region, by virtue of which the sensory portion of the erection reflex arc is blocked out."*

A limp dick (hence the title) or limp whatever name one wants to use in place of penis.

The working definition, however, is a little more complicated, reflecting that the problem usually isn't just a function of soft or hard, but often grades in between. One definition states that potency is a penis hard enough to penetrate a vagina. Another similar definition states that a man is potent if he can engage in successful intercourse.

I'm not sure exactly what either one of those definitions means. I don't really consider being able, with considerable effort and lubricant, to push a mushy penis into a gaping vagina to be what the authors of the first definition really meant by "penetration." And even when a penis has successfully penetrated a vagina, what constitutes "successful intercourse"? From the man and his penis's point of view there is considerable difference between your penis hanging on for dear life or firmly going where he is directed.

I suspect that potency defies a good definition. Potency is when you and your partner can look at each other and say, "That was good," or at least, "That was okay." For many I imagine, potency pre-prostatectomy and post-prostatectomy probably won't be the same thing. It's your call.

Continence:

Webster's: "Ability to refrain from a bodily activity [in this case, urinating]."

Dorland's: "The ability to refrain from yielding to desire. Urinary continence – The ability to retain the contents of the bladder until conditions are proper for urination."

Basically, not peeing your pants.

Prostate (gland):

Webster's: "A firm partially glandular body about the base of the mammalian male urethra."

Dorland's: "A gland which in the male surrounds the neck of the bladder and the urethra. It consists of a median lobe and two lateral lobes, and is made up partly of glandular matter, the ducts from which empty into the prostatic portion of the urethra, and partly of muscular fibers which encircle the urethra."

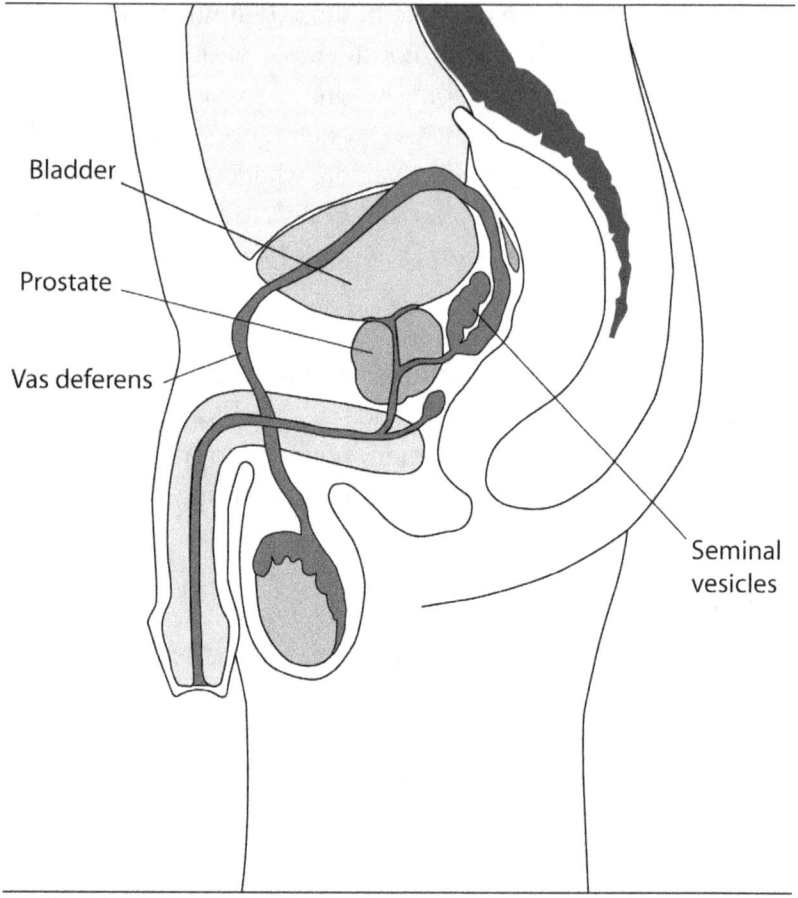

Figure 1 - The prostate gland sits immediately below the bladder and immediately adjacent to the rectum. From the diagram it is apparent that the prostate is surrounded on all sides by lots of important things– which makes surgical access extremely difficult. (created by Mr. Rach Tieszen)

In an adult male, try to imagine something about the size and consistency of a reddish-brown, meaty, tennis ball. On occasion the prostate can grow into something more like a hard lumpy grapefruit in size. Take a look again at the cover that illustrates an actual resected prostate (mine to be exact) in appropriate proportions to the hand.

Dear-Sainted-Wife (DSW):

My DSW and I have been married for forty years. For you, the reader, your DSW may be nether saintly or wifely. When I use the DSW term in the text, what I'm really saying is someone who is at least a partner or friend who can lend both moral and physical support. It might be just a friend to share the bad news of a prostate biopsy, or a more intimate friend to help with the post-prostatectomy catheter plumbing for the first time. The sexual side of the DSW is a partner who is willing to stand by you when things don't go right for the first, or second, or nth time. This is the partner who bucks you up when your male ego is gushing a leak on to the floor (either figuratively or literally).

Surviving a prostatectomy certainly can be done without a DSW, but it is a whole lot easier with one.

Me:

I'm a sixty-year-old white male. I have been happily married to DSW for forty years. We have two grown children who undoubtedly will blush upon reading this and possibly henceforth not acknowledge me in public. I suspect that had my father written this I might have both avoided reading it and moved to another state. Or, hopefully, all of us as children will realize that our parents are, and will continue to be, sexual beings.

Although I have now completely extricated myself from my practice, I have been both a general and forensic pathologist for thirty years. Where individual medical specialists splash around in their own pools of medical expertise, pathologists just dip our toes, but often not too deep, into most all of these specialty pools. Like so many other physicians, I have always thought that bad diseases, particularly cancer, were a diagnosis only to be inflicted on others. But in truth it seems that, diagnostically, "What goes around comes around."

Before the Change

I DON'T BELIEVE I ever really thought that I was bullet-proof. Well, maybe, when I was in my twenties and thirties. At that age you know that somewhere, sometime, there "may" be a bullet with your name on it, but it seems more like a theoretical construct. But by the time you make it to your mid-fifties your bullet has either found you or you are perfectly aware that it is out there somewhere, lurking, but in flight. Yet I guess that by the time I made fifty-five, after either not seeing or dodging a bullet, I believed that the bullet I knew was coming now might reasonably be expected to wait for another ten years, or more.

It's not that I have been perfectly healthy all of my life; at a young age I had an aortic coarctation (a congenital narrowing of my aorta in my chest) repaired, but that was long ago and I was left with no aftereffects. There have been a couple of hernia repairs, and in my forties there was a scary episode of hepatitis that came and went – a bullet dodged.

My cholesterol and blood lipid levels have become a little elevated, but like many (most?) physicians, I successfully self-medicated with the standard statin medication. I was doing the prescribed blood tests to monitor the statin therapy and once, at about age fifty-five, I checked my prostate specific antigen (PSA) level *(more about PSA as a prostate cancer screening test later)*. That particular PSA result was less than 1 – well below the "average" for my age – another bullet dodged, or so I thought.

Like most physicians, I am a big believer in preventive medicine – for you, not me. The DSW had been hounding me for years to get a thorough physical exam. During that time I had pointed out that, as a private pilot, was I getting a "Federally Mandated" physical exam every two years in order to keep my license. Although in my heart of hearts I knew that the FAA physical wasn't really capable of detecting much beyond life-threatening illness, I kept that part to myself – bulletproof.

Then the time came to retire from my general pathology practice and subsequently sell the airplane that I had used to visit far-flung hospitals scattered throughout the expanses of South Dakota, Iowa, and Nebraska. At the time it hadn't dawned on me that I had also sold my excuse for not getting a proper physical exam.

Defenseless, or at least excuse-less, the DSW pounced. I didn't really put up much of a fight. Perhaps I was unconsciously smelling cordite from a gun putting a bullet in flight. The DSW had been getting her annual physicals from an internist I knew and respected; in fact, he had been a resident in our department before he decided to switch gears and go into internal medicine. Most of my partners used him, which lent even more credence to picking him for this, my first official and appropriately thorough physical exam in decades.

Let's call this internist "Bob." Ordinarily he wouldn't warrant a naming, but he comes up later in the story, so "Bob" he is. I had known Bob for years, but I guess I never had really looked at the man. As one of my partners that also went to Bob pointed out, "Have you ever looked at the size of his fingers before?"

Well, no, I never actually had looked at the size of Bob's fingers, but well aware of what he was going to be doing with at least one (it had better be only one) of those fingers, I surreptitiously looked closely the next time I saw Bob in the doctors' lounge. Bob is a big man and his fingers are giant sausages when viewed in the context of where they are going to end up. Bob's digits were not at all similar to the bony little fingers of the guy who had done the FAA physicals before.

As it turned out, Bob, despite his large finger, was very quick and gentle. But, as an aside, for everyone that has had a medicinal finger stuck up their ass, the end of the discomfort doesn't come after the finger is withdrawn. I, for one, am very grateful that these medical practitioners use a lubricating jelly, but what to do with the jelly aftermath is an embarrassing problem. Some docs wipe it off for you. At the time I really couldn't imagine anything much more ego-stripping than standing bent over an exam table while someone else wipes your butt. More thoughtfully, you might be handed a fistful of tissues and then have to decide whether you want to wipe later, forcing you to either stand -- or worse, sit -- through the rest of the exam with a greasy asshole, or wipe it off then and there by yourself while the doc tries to look elsewhere and not overtly judge your wiping technique. No matter what choice you take, inevitably there is a need for a little "touch-up" after the exam is finished.

Back to the story. The touchy-feely part of the exam was perfectly normal, including a prostate that felt normal to a beefy finger. The blood tests, however, were another story. The blood lipids, and those other arcane things that physicians order and no one really knows what they are or why they were ordered, were also perfectly normal. The PSA test however was 3.8 (I won't bother you with units, it just complicates things).

A 3.8 PSA, for my age group, actually was within the "normal" range (the concept of "normal," which I knew as a pathologist, is a somewhat arbitrary construct). As Bob pointed out however, it wasn't so much that my PSA was 3.8 that bothered him, but rather that over three years it had gone from less than 1 to 3.8. That "velocity" of change was not normal. It was Bob's opinion that I needed to see a urologist -- did I have one in mind? Well, as a matter of fact, I did (see below) and the appointment was made.

3 []

I need to insert a couple more asides here. The first: how was it that I already knew which urologist to pick? I have to admit, one of the perks of being a physician is the knowing of how other physicians practice. As a pathologist, my interaction with surgeons primarily was talking with them about the tissue diagnosis of cases they were about to operate on, patients they had operated on, and doing frozen sections while they were actually doing surgery (a technique that allows the pathologist to make a tissue diagnosis in minutes rather than the usual days). Through these interactions between pathologist and surgeons, the pathologist can gain a sense of those surgeons that have a ready grasp of how to therapeutically handle the various diagnostic information we give them. Likewise, the surgeons gain an understanding of which pathologists are good at diagnosing different kinds of lesions.

And through this constant interaction between surgeons and pathologists, the pathologists often get keyed into the scuttlebutt of which surgeons are good at doing certain procedures. Thus, from years of keeping my ear to the professional ground, so to speak, I did indeed know exactly which urologist I wanted to see.

For those of you not so blessed to have this insight into who would be the best urologist (or any specialty for that matter) you must first put at least some trust in the judgment of your referring physician. But I wouldn't stop there. Ask around. As I said at the beginning, prostate cancer is common. It shouldn't be too difficult to find someone you know that has already gone through the process. Seek them out and ask what they thought of their doctor. By and large, prestigious institutions will have better surgeons, but remember that those prestigious institutions train the physicians who staff the perhaps lesser-known medical centers where you might live.

Be ready to ask a designated urologist how many procedures he or she has done. Ask what his (while I admit it might be a "her," but to be honest, there really aren't too many female urologists out there) complication rates are. The national "average" success and complications rates are good to know, but what you really **need** to know is how many procedures that might be done to you your candidate urologist has done (I would like to see several hundred) and what is their individual success and complication rate.

The next short, but necessary, aside is needed to better understand the beginnings of the end of my prostate. What is the PSA (Prostate Specific Antigen)? As the name implies, it is a complex protein manufactured only in the prostate gland. Sorry ladies, your PSA levels are zero, and hopefully I, no longer possessing a prostate, will also continue to have an undetectable PSA level. Normal prostate glands liberate PSA into the blood. If you have a prostate you have a measurable PSA level. The usefulness of the PSA test is that malignant prostate gland cells (usually) liberate more PSA into the blood than benign gland cells. It is unfortunate, however, that the more malignant and aggressive prostate cancer cells can lose their ability to make PSA. Men with these high-grade tumors may therefore not be caught with PSA screening.

In addition to some prostate tumors not secreting PSA, PSA also suffers as a screening test because as the prostate becomes larger – benign prostatic hyperplasia (or BPH) – it dumps more PSA into the blood. The so-called "normal" PSA therefore will be in the 1-2 range in younger men and may approach 5-6 for older men with larger prostates. For a man with a PSA of 4, there is no way to differentiate on the basis of the PSA alone whether the PSA is coming from a small cancer or a benign enlarged prostate.

As I mentioned above, one way to decide whether a borderline PSA is worrisome or not is to see how fast it has been rising over time; obviously this is useful only if there are repeat values to look at. A borderline PSA associated with a definitively enlarged prostate would be less worrisome. A prostate with a distinct lump or nodule, versus a diffusely lumpy-bumpy gland, as felt by doctor's sausage fingers, is worrisome regardless of the PSA level.

Okay, so where was I? Ah yes, my PSA was borderline high in the face of a not spectacularly enlarged prostate and had increased rapidly over the preceding five years. Dr. Bob, bless his heart, had preemptively made the urology appointment and left me to contemplate my fate, for as we all know, when dealing with physician appointments there always is considerable time between when an appointment is made and when it actually happens.

And how exactly did I spend that time? The obvious answer - in denial. The first manifestation of that denial, the first arrow in the physician's quiver of "I don't believe this," was to blame it on lab error. The irony of that situation of course is that pathologists are the ones that oversee clinical labs and who have to wearily listen to other physicians trying to pass off their mistakes as our lab errors. Ironic or not, however, the shoe was now on the other foot and I promptly had my PSA retested.

On retesting, the PSA was 4.1. As a laboratorian, I knew, statistically, there was no significant difference between a 3.8 and a 4.1. The fact that the level had nevertheless actually gone UP was a torpedo below the waterline of my denial battleship. I would like to think that a retested PSA of 3.6 wouldn't have slowed the inevitable, but who knows. Denial is a powerful unmotivator.

Stripped of a "lab error" defense, I spent the next couple of weeks trying vainly to convince myself that the PSA levels could be completely explained by a large prostate, which was actually possible. BPH can (ignore the rarely part) occur somewhat quickly to explain a rapidly rising PSA. Hold that thought!

As a pathologist, however, I routinely dealt with denial lesions: small pea-sized bumps on the skin that their denying owners allowed to grow into grapefruits (you may notice as the story progresses, pathologists have long been known for describing tumors and other pathologic processes with food references) before someone finally got the patient to consider getting the grossly ulcerated foul-smelling thing taken off.

No sir, I wasn't going to let that happen to me. I was going to face this thing head-on. It was indeed "possible" that my PSA values "might" mean that I had prostate cancer, maybe.

I'm going to call my urologist "Jack," perhaps short for "Kojak," a TV star now known only to those of us of a certain age. Jack, like Kojak, shaves his head, which is one of the things he and I have in common. The first appointment with Jack went exactly as I had envisioned it. The waiting room was filled with old men -- well, at least filled with men older than me. That, I presumed, was a good sign -- after all, my Mr. Denial was saying, "You're too young for prostate cancer, just look around."

Jack, however, was well associated with Mr. Denial. To Jack's credit, he made it clear that he was going to treat me as if I wasn't a physician. Not that we didn't immediately do the physician-to-physician collegiality thing of calling each other by our first names. You see, if one doctor calls another physician "Doctor," it either means that the first one really, really, respects the one being addressed, or more likely, is using "Doctor" in a somewhat dismissive way, as a staff physician would address a resident. Anyway, we were Brad and Jack, and he gave me the straight scoop (which I had carefully researched prior to the visit – don't we just love testing our physicians?).

Jack acknowledged all of Mr. Denial's explanations for the rapidly rising PSA levels, and then he lowered the hammer. "You know, Brad, while it is entirely possible your PSA is coming from BPH, I'm frankly worried that you have a small cancer. We could just wait and see what happens, but I don't think you want to live not knowing what's going on. I think we should do a biopsy, don't you?"

Well, actually, at that exact moment there was a small voice in the dark recesses of my mind saying, "Yes, yes, I can live with not knowing! Let's get the hell out of here." The voice that actually spoke however said, "Yeah, let's do it." And "it" was scheduled.

Prior to walking into Jack's office, as a pathologist, I had examined thousands of prostate biopsies under the microscope. I had looked at thousands of little cores of tissue each about a sixteenth of an inch wide and about an inch long. The reassuring thing was than the vast majority of them ended up being benign. Mr. Denial was once again revving his engines.

The flip side of most prostate biopsies being negative was that when a urologist is truly concerned, they don't just give up with one set of negative biopsies (by a "set" I mean usually six to twelve, or more, pieces of tissue taken in one "biopsy" session – usually from the top, middle, and bottom of the prostate on each side). Well aware that any given biopsy session actually samples no more than a tenth of a percent of the actual prostate volume, the urologist will often keep plugging (pun intended) along with biopsies every six months or so until they eventually find a cancer, which usually takes no more than a couple of years. So there, Mr. Denial, even if the biopsy is negative, Jack is going to keep looking until he finds the cancer he is concerned is there and which I'm trying, unsuccessfully, to not worry about.

A few weeks of smoldering concern, often forcibly pushed from my mind, passed. The funny thing is, that despite the large number of men who must be having their prostate biopsied, I hadn't actually talked to anyone about having the procedure done. Even those men I had talked to who have had their prostates taken out, and who must have had biopsies, hadn't said a word about the procedure. I didn't have a clue what to expect. Was that a good sign or a bad one?

While waiting for the scheduled biopsy I had the good fortune of enduring another colonoscopy. Well, actually, as many of you know, the colonoscopy itself is easy; fun, perhaps – they inject pleasantly mind-numbing drugs into you, you awake feeling still pleasantly buzzed, and you get to go home, missing work, while other colonoscopy non-initiates feel just a tad sorry for you. The colonoscopy prep, however, is a bitch worthy of a story in itself. Wouldn't it just be easier, I have wondered, just to pour the damn prep stuff directly into the toilet and avoid the middleman?

The colonoscopy is relevant only because it led to false perceptions about the prostate biopsy. I mean, with the colonoscopy they fill you full of drugs and then stick a big hose up your butt; shouldn't the prostate biopsy be similar? After all, they did say I needed someone to drive me home afterward.

It seems that the only similarity between a colonoscopy and a prostate biopsy is the prep, not the similar part I wanted. I had hoped that perhaps the reason no one ever talks about getting their prostate biopsied was that they didn't remember it – alas, that's not the case. The sorry truth is that there are no mind-numbing drugs used during prostate biopsies – I was there, so to speak, for the whole thing.

At the appointed time a cheerful nurse leads you to a darkened room, instructs you to remove your clothes, and gives you one of those ridiculous gowns that seem somewhat superfluous in a urologist's office. You lie down on a somewhat sparsely padded table and shortly thereafter realize the potential for a new invention – a KY jelly warmer – as a big glop of the stuff is liberally smeared over your prep-abused arse.

Shortly thereafter is a request to "bear down." Bear down on what? – Oh Lord, someone was sticking a baseball bat up my asshole! Later I would describe it as a baseball bat with a porcupine on the end, but that part hadn't quite materialized yet.

Although the prostate can be biopsied through the skin behind the scrotum, the preferred method, as you may have guessed, is directing a biopsy needle forward from inside the rectum. This used to be done by hand – a somewhat barbaric procedure which I had witnessed long ago, but which now is done via the just inserted semi-automated "baseball bat."

Part of the baseball bat is an ultrasound probe that Jack reassuringly told me was showing a picture of a normal prostate. While that was good sign, because prostate cancer usually doesn't produce a "bad" ultrasound until it is quite extensive, the vast majority of cancerous prostates unfortunately have normal ultrasounds. I don't think Mr. Denial even stirred with the good ultrasound news.

While the rectal mucosa is less sensitive to being poked than skin, it still hurts. Therefore, the first part of the procedure is injecting some Novocaine (or its equivalent) into the mucosa and around the prostate. This also is accomplished via the baseball bat. While these injections were being made, Jack asked me how things were going. Without thinking, I said, "It's okay, it just feels like a little prick." There was a moment of silence eventually broken by a giggle from Jack's nurse. What?? – Oh shit! Jack actually thought it was quite funny too, and went on to tell a story about an obstetrician ready to inject an about-to-deliver lady with some anesthetic. She was told that she would feel just "a small prick," to which she replied, "That's what got me in here in the first place."

The biopsy needles are also part of the baseball bat – the porcupine part. They were more than a "small prick"; more like the kind of pain that you take a deep breath to tolerate and hope it doesn't last too long – which it doesn't. It wasn't a pleasurable experience, but tolerable. At the conclusion of the procedure there was again that awkward moment of what to do with a greasy butt. And although they warned me, the amount of bloodstaining on what I was left to wipe away was somewhat disconcerting. There also was a warning about possible blood in the urine (which didn't happen) and bloody semen (which did happen and was a shock to all involved). Although I think I could have driven home afterward, I suppose that being violated by a baseball bat equivalent and left bloody after the exchange would potentially be distracting for one's driving – yah think?

For years I have been diagnosing tissue biopsies and have abstractly thought of what my diagnoses would mean to those people behind the named but otherwise anonymous tissue requisitions. Professionally I was the dispenser of joyful (benign) and calamitous (malignant) news. The shoe was decidedly on the other foot now.

I had decided that I didn't want the members of my former group to be the first to know whether or not I had cancer. Therefore, I elected to let Jack send the biopsy material out to the pathology group he usually used. In retrospect, that might have been a mistake.

Physicians for years have been telling patients after a biopsy that there will be a wait (usually several days) while the tissue is processed in pathology. This undoubtedly has led many patients to believe that we pathologists are cruelly insensitive to their agony of waiting for a result. That's not true. The truth is, most of the time spent waiting for a biopsy result comes from getting the tissue to the pathologist and the results back to the physician rather than the actual diagnostic process in pathology. It can be done quickly. Had my biopsy tissue been sent to my old group, I would have had an answer the afternoon of the next day; as it was, I was forced to wait a week. For those that have waited for a possible cancer diagnosis, you know full well, a week is a very, very, long time to wait.

During that week I tried to convince myself that by dint of pure willing it to be, I could make the biopsy benign, with the corollary being that even entertaining thoughts that it might be malignant would make it so. I was, by the day appointed for the results to return, outwardly calm and internally more than a little frazzled. The "diagnosis day" dragged on with no call from Jack's office. Finally, around 4:00 p.m. the phone rang with Jack's office on the caller ID.

While diagnosing badness for people in years past I had from time to time imagined what "that call" would be like. I think the worst case scenario would have been, "Hello, Mr. Randall. Your biopsy results are in. Could we schedule an appointment for you to see Dr. Jack?"

"Well, okay, but could you tell me what the results are?"

"I'm sorry, Mr. Randall, but you will have to wait to talk to Dr. Jack about that."

I have always thought that the above would be cruel and unusual punishment. And it's not what happened to me. The call came from Jack's nurse and it was short and to the point. "Dr. Randall, the biopsy report has come back and it shows a malignancy. Can you and your wife come in tomorrow to discuss the results with Dr. Jack?" I've never worked in an office that sees patients, but I still find it amazing that one can get non-emergent appointments for the next day.

Well, there I was with the phone still in my hand. Damn, even with a week to prepare, and a week's worth of actively denying that this day would come, it still was a shock. I mean, cancer is something other people, older people get. Shit!

DSW had seen the caller ID and knew full well who had called and with what news. Nearly forty years of living with someone obviated the need for words when I plodded up the basement stairs. Nevertheless, the question had to be asked, "Is it..?"

"Yes."

"Oh..."

The rest of that day remains a little foggy. There were a few tears that ultimately transformed into quiet "poor-little-old-me" moments on my part. I guess that experience living with me gave DSW the knowledge of knowing exactly when to pull the plug on my wallowing.

Sometime later that day the "buck-up buddy" message began. After all, let's put this in perspective, it's "only" prostate cancer. That "only" hurt to hear, but it was true. *Because of PSA tests and prostatectomies, the mortality from prostate cancer has dramatically dropped, which isn't true for the ugly cancers out there like cancers of the breast and lung and pancreas and liver and brain along, with the host of lymphomas and leukemias.* To her credit, she didn't actually say that I was "lucky" to have only prostate cancer, but the message was received.

There continued to be, and continue to be, dark moments; the "Why me?" moments. But at least they aren't "This sucker is going to kill me" moments. What I had instead were "This is going to do bad things to me" moments. These are things that as a physician I already knew on an intellectual level and was rapidly relearning on a personal, visceral, level.

Prostate cancer is one of the rare cancers where the treatment for the cancer may well be worse than no treatment at all. If a man makes it to eighty years old or more and is diagnosed with prostate cancer, the odds are overwhelming that he will die "with," but not "of," his disease. When did that eighty-year-old's cancer begin? Who knows? But for many men it began years, if not decades, earlier. So then, how do you know what cancer in a younger man is going to just sit there and grow indolently for years, and which is going to grow beyond the prostate gland, metastasize to bone and elsewhere, and kill you? The answer, unfortunately, remains, "Who knows?"

So that was the crap shoot that faced me and the thousands of other men in the past, and most likely for some time in the future, who will need to decide what to do once their prostate goes "bad." On the one hand, you could simply do nothing. If I was a seventy-something man, that is probably what I would have done; were I in my late sixties – maybe. Fifty-eight, now that's a real gamble. Do nothing at fifty-eight and there is a real serious risk of letting the horse out of the barn – which is problematic, since it is difficult to know when the horse has left and nearly impossible to repair once the barn door is found open and the horse gone.

On the other hand, surgical or radiation therapy for prostate cancer has well-known, and very real, risks of significant side effects. There is a smoldering low level of very severe risk with either procedure – dying, turning into a vegetable, perforating a bowel, that sort of thing. Those are the sorts of things that are so rare that we don't really think about them when we are signing the permission slip.

It's the other risks that grab a man's attention. A very real chance exists, perhaps not up to fifty percent, but close, that treatment for prostate cancer will produce some degree of incontinence or impotence; and that, let me tell you, does grab a man's attention.

So what do you do? Do you take an unquantifiable risk of doing nothing, knowing that if you are wrong it might kill you? Or do you opt for more aggressive therapy that quite likely will remove most, hopefully all, of the cancer and then deal with a high likelihood of significant complications, i.e., a very important part of you not working properly?

As I have stated above, there is no "right" answer to that question. Even though as a physician I was already reasonably up to date with the relevant medical literature, like everyone else facing this decision, it was time to do some Internet research. Don't expect to answer your questions solely from surfing the Web. The problem isn't that you won't find enough information; quite the opposite.

There is way, way, too much on the Web. Every possible treatment option has its advocates and statistics to back it up. Remember, as statisticians and pollsters will tell you, data can be either manufactured or badly twisted to support nearly any point of view. If you are looking for some magic wand to separate the wheat from the chaff of data overload on the Web, it doesn't exist.

Nevertheless, I believe that it is important to be as well informed as possible prior to that first "Okay-now-you have-cancer, what-are-we-going-to-do-about-it" talk with your urologist. Listen very carefully to what the urologist has to say -- after all, he does this for a living and theoretically, at least, should know more about your options that you do. On the other hand, also be aware of his inherent biases. There is very little motivating a urologist to send all of his prostate cancer patients either home to do nothing or to the radiation therapist.

A very important part of the decision-making process is dependent on the trust you are willing to place in any physician. Does he seem to know what he is doing? Does he appear to be confident in his surgical skills? Can you clearly understand, and believe, in what he is saying? These are ambiguous yardsticks which may or may not reflect on a urologist's skill, but which are critically important for that level of trust that is necessary between a patient and a physician. May be it's just me, but I have always felt that patients that trust their physicians do better.

Jack did a great job with that first visit. It was clear that he had done this first cancer therapy presentation many times before, without it sounding stale. I think I did throw him off his game a little, however, as he admitted - spelling everything out to a fellow physician was something a little new to him. As he freely admitted, Jack really hadn't worked with a patient that actually saw and handled prostates perhaps more than he did. But his surgical techniques were undoubtedly a little more precise than mine. Jack solved the doctor-to-doctor dilemma by starting out with, "Brad, I know that you undoubtedly know more about prostate cancer therapy than my usual patient, but it is easier if I don't talk to you as a physician, but rather give you the same talk I would give any patient." That was fine with me, and very much appreciated by DSW, who wanted to hear what her husband was up against.

From what I knew, I thought Jack gave a very balanced review of my treatment options. Doing nothing was not a viable option – I was just too young. Radiation *was* a viable option, but the down side was that fewer complications earlier was balanced with a greater likelihood of complications later and the difficulty of treating recurrent cancer in a pre-irradiated field (might a radiation therapist have spun this a little differently? – perhaps, but that's where the "trust" thing came in).

The type of prostate cancer I had also entered into the treatment equation. As I well knew, for many years pathologists have been assigning a Gleason's score to prostate cancer. In its most common usage, the pathologist assigns a score of 1 to 5 for the most common pattern of the tumor and again for the worst part of the tumor and then adds those two numbers. As it turns out, scores of 2 to 4 rarely, if ever, happen. Therefore, scores of 5-6 are considered relatively "low" grade, 7-8 of "moderate" grade, and 9-10 are considered "high" grade tumors.

The bad news was that my tumor scored out as a 7. The good news was that it wasn't a 9. The other bit of good news was that the tumor appeared to be confined just to the bottom part of the left side of the prostate. The pathologist that reviewed my biopsy estimated that no more than 5% of the prostate was malignant. (Mr. Denial would insist that I personally review the microscopic slides from the biopsy. There was that itsy-bitsy non-rational hope that the outside pathologist had blown it, which of course was nonsense. When I did look at the slides I saw that his Gleason's score was perhaps a little generous on the light side. I might have called it an 8. There also was some suggestion of possible peri-neural tumor invasion, which just like it sounds, isn't a good thing.)

The small amount of prostate involved argued for a less aggressive treatment like radiation. The higher grade of tumor, however, suggested the need for more aggressive therapy: surgery.

Jack argued that surgical removal of the prostate gland was the best course for me. But the decision didn't end there. Exactly what type of surgical treatment? A few years ago there was only one option, the retropubic radical prostatectomy where the surgeon made a large incision just below (the "retro" part) of the pubic bone and tunneled down under the bladder and with the usual surgical instruments carefully removed the prostate gland. Once the prostate was gone, the bottom of the bladder and the resected end of the urethra (the channel that drains the urine from the bladder to the end of the penis) were sewn back together. For its advocates, the retropubic prostatectomy allowed the surgeon to directly visualize the prostate and the tissue that surrounded it to make sure any obvious tumor was removed. The surgeon was also able to sample the lymph nodes of the pelvis to make sure that there was no metastatic tumor. The lymph nodes were examined by the pathologist during the surgery by a process called "frozen section." During my career I have looked at a lot of these lymph nodes and have only rarely, very rarely, seen one that was positive.

The real problem with the retropubic prostatectomy is that it forces the surgeon to work in a very confined space where it is both difficult to see and even more difficult to manipulate his surgical instruments (see Figure 1 again back in the Glossary). This difficult work space creates risks for damaging neighboring structures like the rectum and bladder, along with the possibilities of a leaky connection between the bladder and the urethra.

Yet good urologists in most cases could avoid those more adverse risks. The real problem however is that the nerves that control an erection travel in a delicate, loose network that immediately surrounds the outside of the prostate. To precisely separate these nerves away from the prostate was a far more complex task for the urologist. The urologist was faced with balancing nerve sparing against adequate resection. It is a difficult balancing act, since no urologist wants to leave cancer behind. As a result, despite their best efforts, urologists that did open retropubic prostatectomies found that a very high percent of their patients had postoperative impotence.

The next advance was the laparoscopic prostatectomy. Instead of having to fit his beefy hands into a small artificial space beneath the bladder, the urologist now could send a flexible tube, or series of tubes, into this confined area. The operative tools and visualization were all carried in via snakes about the size of your thumb. The result was it was easier to work in a small space with smaller tools.

And no sooner was laparoscopic surgery catching on than the next, and currently hot, surgical advance leapt onto the prostatectomy stage – robotic surgery. (Fig. 2) Now, the urologist doesn't even have to get his gloves dirty. Unlike laparoscopic surgery where the surgeon still had to manipulate what was happening at the ends of the laparoscopes by hand, with robotic surgery an intermediary has been inserted.

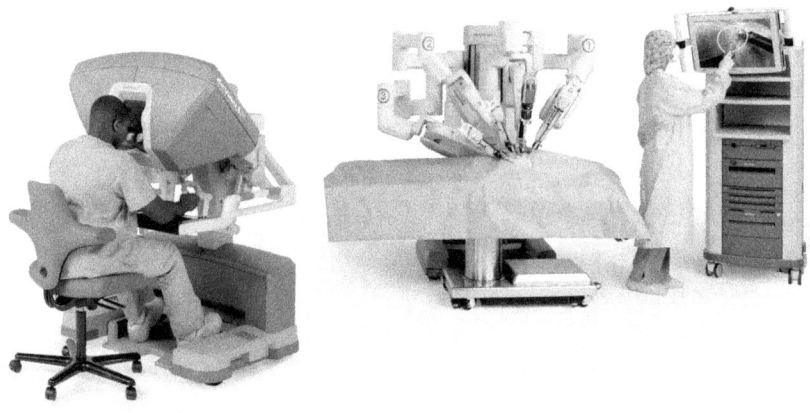

Figure 2 - A representation of the da VinciTM Surgical System used for robotic prostatectomies. The surgeon seen sitting at his console on the left controls the robotic arms hovering over the patient in the center frame. (Used by permission from Intuitive Surgical Inc.)

Just to make things clear, a "robot" does not do "robotic" surgery. The "robot" is a device that translates small motions of the urologist's hands that have been inserted into a glove-like device (minus the small "shakes" inherent in all of us) into tiny, very precise motions at the end of small manipulators that have been inserted through the abdominal wall and into the virtual peri-prostatic space. The "robot" allows the surgeon to make precise movements less than a millimeter long without the shakiness inherent in even the steadiest surgeon's hand.

The theory is that such precise, delicate resection techniques will allow the urologist to deftly separate nerve from prostate, allowing preservation of erectile function while at the same time assuring complete tumor resection. It is a lofty claim, and it is unclear if it is true. It certainly seems to make sense and has driven robotic prostatectomy into the preferred and most performed prostatectomy technique. As one urologist complained recently, "If as a urologist you aren't doing robotic surgery, you soon will find yourself not doing prostatectomies" (which is a big part of any urology practice).

Testimonials to robotic surgery abound on the Internet urology websites and elsewhere. The hard information is less convincing. One oft-quoted study showed little difference in long-term complications between open prostatectomy and the other procedures – and before you say it – the obvious problem with that study was that it combined laparoscopic and robotic surgery into one group. The study however did clearly indicate that compared to the retropubic prostatectomy, either the laparoscopic or robotic procedures had their patients more quickly out of the hospital, more quickly recuperated, and with fewer immediate post-operative complications.

This is how I sifted through the chaff and wheat of the robotic or nonrobotic controversy. First, you have to remember that with the exception of those few new urologists coming out into practice for the last few years, none of the "more experienced" urologists had any experience whatsoever with robotic surgery before it became available. Those practicing urologists therefore had to go out and learn this new procedure. And its no surprise that at the beginning of their learning curve their success rates weren't as good as they were later. The data on whether robotic surgery lives up to its hype therefore is corrupted by the experience level of those doing the surgery.

I realize that this experience thing puts the urologists on the early side of the learning curve in a "Catch-22" situation. They can't get better without doing more procedures, and they can't get more procedures because they are just getting started. Dr. Urologist, I feel your pain, I really do, because it's what every physician goes through when they start. Nevertheless, when it came to my particular prostate, I wanted a veteran.

How do you know a veteran urologist? Part of that answer comes from keeping your ear to the ground around the hospital. In my case it was watching the flow of surgical specimens through the pathology department and listening to the surgeons' chatter when we dealt with them. Obviously, most people don't have that kind of access, but your referring physician should have some idea who's better and who's not. Just ask your referring physician who they would go to if it was their, or their family's, prostate on the line.

Ultimately you just have to ask your urologist what his experience is. How many cases? How many had recurrences? What is his complication rate? Follow up on the complication rates. Don't just ask how many of his patients leaked after the surgery, but how much and for how long? It's great to know how many could grow an erection after the surgery, but how many more could a year, or two years, afterward? And make sure you personalize it. If your urologist is sufficiently experienced, he should be able to answer your questions not only in general, but more specifically for how much and what kind of cancer you have. Bottom line – how much is enough experience? That's a tough call, but personally, I was looking for at least 200-300 robotic surgeries total, and around 30-40 or more per year.

Ultimately I did elect to go with the robotic surgery. Jack, perhaps more openly than he would have been for a nonphysician patient, offered to send me to the Mayo Clinic (substitute here whatever super-brand name medical center you wish) for the surgery. I turned him down. One, because I deemed that he did indeed have the level of experience I wanted. Two, even the mega-centers can screw up. And three, experience eventually carries you only so far. After a time any procedure becomes a "meat-and-potatoes" operation. I would go to the mega-center for fancy French cooking, but given the ubiquitousness of prostate surgery, robotic prostatectomies have become a "meat-and-potatoes" operation.

And why did I elect to go with the robotic procedure? That really was never a question. Once I ruled out the more conservative radiation treatment, there wasn't really an option. It seems that even though the superiority of the robotic procedure hasn't been completely validated, that's essentially all you can find any urologist willing to do.

I thought Jack did a very good job with the "what-to-do" decision-making process. He spelled the options out, literally on several pieces of paper, and sent DSW and me home to think things over. It was my prostate, my decision -- but DSW was supportive, not just passively, but with helping to tease the arguments out – the pros and cons of what to do. I truly do not believe that the consequences of the sexual politics of our family even entered her mind during these deliberations, as they most clearly did for me. She made it clear she understood the consequences of what I was deciding, and she made it clear that she could live with it, and therefore so could I.

It was pretty clear to me upon leaving Jack's office after that first post-cancer visit what I was going to do. I mean, after all, what else exactly had I been thinking about from the moment I saw the first elevated PSA level? There could be no doubt, by the time we saw Jack a couple of days later, that the decision had been exceptionally well-vetted. Jack would do a robotic prostatectomy on me. The date and time were set. The finality was akin to hearing the judge's gavel fall in a courtroom.

From the moment I walked out of that office, there was a dark little voice whispering in the back of my mind, "What the fuck did you just do to yourself?" The answer of course was, "The right thing." And I believed, and continue to believe, in that answer. Nevertheless, even now, I still hear, and wonder about, that dark little question.

The next several weeks were a time of pretending all was normal. The news quickly got out and there were days of acknowledging little condolence speeches from friends and colleagues, all of which dissipated rather rapidly once, the expressions of regret having been said, there was nothing more to do than go back to normality.

After an inexplicable delay my biopsy slides finally arrived for my review. They provided some closure, and (as I alluded to above), provided some slightly more ominous news that helped to reinforce my treatment decision.

The week before the surgery DSW and I went to Florida. Sun, and beach, and friends – life goes on. The prospect of the impending surgery hovered sub rosa during the trip and intruded openly only once; consider the incongruous image of me walking on the sand with a cell phone to my ear while being taken step by step through the pre-admission pre-op questionnaire. "Religious preference?" – whoops, don't step on that shell – "Emergency contact person?" – look out for that wave – "Who will drive you home?" – My God, that's a beautiful – bikini...that's not fair, don't even think about that...what was the question? "Dietary preferences?"

The days marched on until the weekend before the surgery, which had been scheduled for early Monday (one of the things people that work in hospitals learn is that surgeries should always be scheduled early in the week – have your surgery on Thursday or Friday and when you are having troubles on the second post-op day you'll end up talking to your surgeon's partner on call while the guy you really want to be talking to is enjoying the back nine).

It was the first weekend in April. Sunday dawned clear and a little chilly, proving to be a nice day for a walk. The little overnight bag was ready, since I didn't want to be putting things together before we went to the hospital at some very dark hour in the morning – a time of the day that I would have been perfectly happy to have known only on a theoretical basis. Pre-op dietary restrictions prevented the meal I would have liked to have had, but didn't prevent it from being eaten earlier on Saturday.

I had three goals for that last day of "intactness." One, avoid thinking about tomorrow as much as possible. Two, the "CLF" (see below). And three, the bowel prep that once again was being thrust upon (into?) my poor abused colon. It was important that all three be accomplished in the stated order.

Acronyms hold a special fascination for me; they shorten, befuddle, and confuse. In a medical chart they can drive you to distraction – and I love to make up my own. "CLF," the "Ceremonial Last Fuck." For those of you not willing to wait for the end, it fortunately proved not to be true, but at the time, I wasn't exactly sure of that.

As I mentioned at the beginning, this isn't a "kiss-and-tell" story. The details of the CLF are between me and DSW. It was however a fitting end to one era and the beginning of another. Ironically, the post-biopsy seminal blood had finally cleared.

Hopefully the necessary ordering of that Sunday's events should now be obvious. The colon prep was a "blast."

Operation Day

THEY SAY THAT condemned prisoners usually sleep well the night before their executions. I can't speak to that, but I do know that I slept well the night before my surgery. It is hard in retrospect to know if the emotional numbness that greeted me on Monday was dread, or just being up and about several hours before I usually would have been.

I have always thought that hospitals wanted their surgical patients in early so the surgeons could get done in time to make rounds and see patients in the afternoon. Undoubtedly those scheduling concerns drive the early OR times, but I had never considered that early morning shocking the pre-op patients might also serve a calming, pacifying purpose. I wonder, does cattle slaughtering go better in the early morning?

The one thing you want as a pre-op patient, no matter if you are getting a knee scoped, a prostate removed, or risky brain surgery, is an admission staff that knows exactly what they are doing but which at the same time recognizes that everything is new and more than a bit overwhelming for you. I could say that I was lucky and experienced just such a combination, but I don't think that luck had anything to do with it. Undoubtedly there are some bad apples in the business, but by and large it has been my experience that most hospital employees, but particularly those on the front end of the patient experience, are very good at what they do – a large part of which is making you feel comfortable.

Fill out this form, fill out that form, talk to the nurse, talk to the anesthesiologist, say goodbye to your clothes (you did remember not to bring any valuables, didn't you?). Condemned prisoners may sleep through the night, but I doubt they are quite so calm as the pre-execution hours dwindle into minutes. I wasn't.

As the time got closer, little tendrils of dread and foreboding slowly began to coalesce into an outward flattening of affect and a growing pit in the stomach. I think that the staff had seen my deer in the headlights look before. A newbie nurse might have tried to divert your attention with extraneous chatter; the pro nursing staff just gives you a smile, checks to make sure everything is as okay as it can be, and then leaves you alone. I'm sure DSW understood that also. We just sat in the little prep room, watching but not seeing the TV, and held hands.

Inevitably, in that slow-motion flow of time, a nice lady stuck her head in our little cubicle and said, "It's time." I had a mental image of how things were supposed to go from that point on. A wheelchair would be waiting at the cubicle door which I would ride, regally pushed by my attendants, like a conquering hero, to the operating room. En route I would deign to nod or perhaps even give a small wave to those scrubs-clad workers I encountered. This, I assumed, was the sort of adoration the Mayans, for example, gave to their soon to be sacrificial victims.

As it turned out, the only part of that fantasy that I got right was the sacrificial part. They made me walk to the OR, shuffling along in my hospital slipper/socks, a thin robe to hide the ubiquitous backless hospital gown, while ignominiously pushing an IV pole ahead of me. The blue scrubs wearers either ignored me or looked the other way as another victim passed. I felt like a steer getting a brief tour of the abattoir.

The walk seemed interminable, but eventually my attendant (whom I needed to show me the way, but was she also there to make sure I didn't bolt?) and I turned the corner to my operating room. From time to time

I have been in a variety of ORs, both as a patient and as a physician observer, but I have to admit, this one was, as a music professor friend I know would say, "Way cool!"

The OR was larger than most, but much of the space was taken up by the hulking mass of the "robot" as it lurked in the corner (see Figure 2 again). Like most ORs, the center of the room revolved around the plinth-like table – my table. I tried to push the comparison with my autopsy bench out of my mind.

The patient's final act of ownership with the procedure to come, for those lucky enough to arrive here under their own power, is to accede to the request to, "Please lie down on the table." Being slid off a gurney onto the OR table makes it "their" fault for the OR staff (versus "your" fault if you flub up) if somehow you end up three feet lower than intended. Climbing up there yourself means, "What the fuck am I getting myself into?"

As I'm about to settle down onto this templar bench I realize that it is coated with yellowish goo, akin to something that may have dripped from an *Alien* movie who's monster had a bad cold. However it proved to be neither slimy or gooey, but rather warm and quite comfortable – which was a welcome relief when you were expecting a cold tabletop.

For years I have argued with my dentist that he needs to put something to look at on the ceiling of his exam rooms. From my vantage point I realized that the same principle would apply to ORs too, although unlike the dentist's office, there hopefully would be considerably less ceiling staring time here in the OR. Anonymous mask-covered faces flitted in and out of my vision. Most of these masked heads were murmuring amongst themselves in what I hoped was professional preparation-speak and not a political or sports discussion. Calm voices occasionally penetrated as someone announced a subtle repositioning of body parts and a decommissioning of what little clothing I had taken into the OR.

As I was slowly coming to grips with this surreal dance that surrounded me, a voice from over my head calmly said, "Brad, I'm going to give you a little something to take the edge off." Now let me tell you, from personal experience and from watching this done to others, what this voice meant was, "Brad, lights out." I was just about to say something to the effect, "Yeah, sure, you expect me to believe that?" when what really happened was that I awoke six hours later in a hospital room with DSW hovering overhead.

As I learned later, what I remembered and what actually happened were a little different. Jack and I apparently had a lively preoperative discussion and then once again discoursed in the recovery suite. I would like to believe that I was completely appropriate and didn't give away any secrets or tell horribly lurid jokes, as forensic pathologists on occasion can. He hasn't said and I haven't asked.

In retrospect, several weeks later, I realized that this "going into the OR" thing is a religious metaphor. This is not to espouse any particular religion or religiosity, but just the concept. As a penitent, you enter the temple, stripped of all of your worldly possessions. To enter the temple you must faithfully place your body and soul fully into another's hands; the hands of an unseen god-like presence that you know is hovering nearby. You are rewarded by hushed reverence and support of the temple acolytes. The temple radiates -- no, nearly bursts -- with the message, "Trust us, put your faith in us, and we will heal." Do the people that design and run ORs know this? I hope not. But whatever religion you happen to claim, if any, I don't think they could propose a better send-off from this mortal coil than you'll get in an OR.

The immediate postoperative few days went off more or less as expected. Having had both the traditional abdominal surgery and the endoscopic kind, there is little doubt that there is far less discomfort with the latter. A friend who had the open retropubic type of prostatectomy was nursing an aching belly for days and had to spend four days in the hospital before being sent home.

I spent a night in the hospital (perhaps a little more than twenty-four hours) and was then sent home. In retrospect another night probably wouldn't have been a bad idea, but it wasn't a big deal. I was up walking the same day as the surgery, and avoided the stomach upsets that occasionally can complicate general anesthesia.

By the evening of my surgery, DSW and I had resumed our usual evening cribbage game. She usually wins, but that night I double skunked her. She attributed this to luck, and perhaps she was right, but without any thought I offered this explanation: "Luck had nothing to do with it. People have known for years that a certain percentage of every man's intelligence resides between his legs. I've just had the plug removed and that intelligence has bubbled up where it belongs. You're lucky you were only just double skunked." For what it's worth, that was the last double skunking, on my part, and DSW continues to win more than she loses.

A week after the surgery I was back at work, although the pace did move a little slower than usual. Except for the catheter care (which I will talk about in greater detail below) the surgery and its recovery actually went quite smoothly. Maybe that's telling on myself a bit, because when people found out that I just had undergone a prostatectomy the looks in their eyes suggested a belief that such a surgery must involve horrific surgical atrocities on the body normal and that my seeming good postoperative health must therefore represent incredible pain tolerance and strength of will on my part. I did not dissuade them from that belief. Bottom line, the surgery itself wasn't that big of a deal.

There was however one small postoperative hiccup that I bring up only to tell a story about fleas and cutters. By the third postoperative day my main complaint was a grinding, burning substernal (what some would call the solar plexus) pain. Like a good patient I called my surgeon and relayed my concerns. Like a good surgeon he asked me about other more surgical related pains but could offer no explanation for what I was suffering. In so doing, he acted as a "cutter."

"Cutters" were, back in the day, the barbers of the medical world: largely uneducated in the art and science of medicine, but good at wielding a sharp knife. The modern day cutters obviously are our surgeons and those other medical specialists that use scalpels as a part of their practice (most urologists fall into this camp while the OB/GYNs may or may not).

Those physicians who don't regularly cut people as part of their practice are the group that coined the "cutter" moniker. The surgeons, on the other hand, refer to their non-cutting brethren as "fleas" (the theory being that these docs are always, like fleas, "jumping from one diagnosis to another"). The "fleas" comprise all of the internal medicine specialties, pediatricians, and psychiatrists. The hospital-based physicians (anesthesiologists, radiologists, and pathologists) don't really fall into either camp – despite my daily use of sharp cutting instruments…I guess your patients have to be alive to count. The fleas have always thought of themselves as smarter than the cutters, and surprisingly, a lot of cutters believe that too.

Anyway, when a cutter is faced with something (like a stomachache) that isn't obviously a surgical problem, their first reaction is to label that a flea issue and wash their hands of the nuisance by referring the patient back to their friendly internist, which is what Jack did.

To be honest, I never really gave Bob a chance. Despite DSW's, and my son the doctor's, assurances that I was wrong, I knew all about that pain in my gut; I had felt it before during a nasty bout of hepatitis. I proceeded then to commit a physician no-no: I diagnosed myself. My gastric stress ulcer had returned. The stress was there, the pain was there – bingo! To confirm the diagnosis I purchased some over-the-counter Pepcid (what is known as a H2 blocker) and two days later the pain was gone – a classical therapeutic trial gone right.

Then, to confirm my diagnosis, and get DSW off my back, I called

Bob, who graciously told me he agreed with both my diagnosis and treatment, although he did prescribe a little more industrial strength H2 blocker that resulted in the complete resolution of the problem. Presented here as a classic case of cutters, fleas, and self-diagnosing physicians.

Of Hoses and Bags

THE MAJOR POSTOPERATIVE nuisance of the prostatectomy (no matter how it is done) is the extended (in my case, two-week) stint with an indwelling urinary catheter. (Fig. 3) The need for a catheter makes sense when you consider the plumbing problems for the urologist. Having removed a couple of inches of the tube (urethra) between the base of the bladder and the end of the penis where the prostate once was, the urologist has to stitch the urethra from the bottom of the prostate back to the bottom of the bladder.

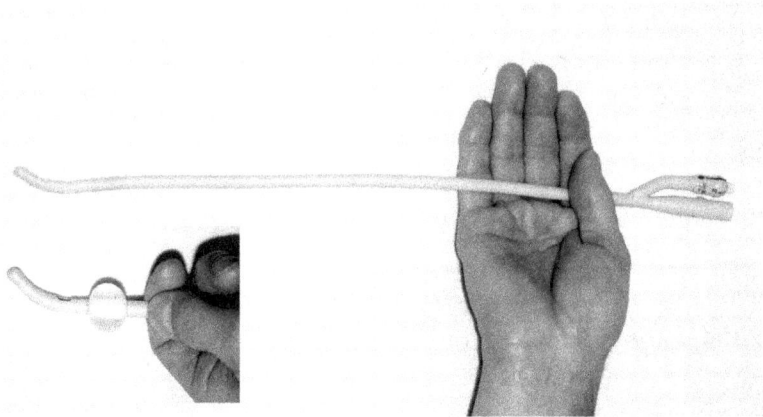

Figure 3 - The Foley catheter. The emptying end and the port to inflate the balloon at the tip are to the left. The insert shows the balloon at the tip inflated and hopefully makes it clear that horrible things happen if an attempt is made to pull the catheter out of the bladder without first deflating the balloon.

By having a catheter in place as a stent, it makes it much easier to sew the ends of the urethra back together. Plus, by having the urine pass through the catheter, there aren't any worries that the suture line anastamosis will leak. The anastamosis line will also heal more quickly without having to deal with the pressures of the patient pushing hard to get done peeing quickly.

So it was no surprise that when I finally awakened enough on that first operative day to lift the sheets up and look at what Jack had wrought, a yellow rubber catheter was snaking out of my little buddy to disappear hopefully into some urine bag attached to the bed. To keep the catheter from coming out, a small balloon at the tip of the catheter in the bladder is inflated with water (see Figure 3 again). Trying to pull a catheter out without deflating this balloon is an extremely uncomfortable experience, and in a post-prostatectomy patient a probable urologic disaster. Even on those days of most intensely loathing my catheter, that thought never, even remotely, went through my mind.

Sometimes the inflated balloon at the tip of the bladder can fool the bladder into thinking you need to pee. This sensation can range from being a little irritating, to driving you "nucking-futs," to gut- wrenching spasms. Fortunately I avoided that problem, which as it turned out was about the only quarter given to me by that diabolical piece of rubber tubing.

Let's get one thing straight, there are catheters and then there are CATHETERS. The sick patient in the hospital that can't pee by themselves gets a little wimpy tube whose only function is to get urine from point A to point B. In post-prostatectomy patients they don't use catheters; they use garden hoses (a urology nurse recently told me to stop whining, saying, "If you think that what you got was a 'garden hose,' you should see the 'fire hose' that could have been used."). As Jack pointed out, this makes sense. The urologist wants as big a stent as possible for the urethral anastamosis because once the catheter/garden hose is gone, the opening it protected is going to contract.

One of the postoperative complications of a prostatectomy is a stricture, or narrowing, of the anastamosis. Sometimes this problem can occur immediately after the catheter is removed and presents as a very, very, uncomfortable man who hasn't been able to pee for way too long and is convinced of an unobtainable need to deliver twins.

The cure is to put a probe back up the urethra and open the narrowing. This sounds like, and is, an unpleasant procedure, but when it results in deflating a bladder the perceived size of a watermelon, it doesn't seem so bad.

Once again I was fortunate, like most post- prostatectomy patients, to avoid that type of acute obstruction. Narrowing of the anastmosis, however, can occur slowly over time and also may need the "rotor-rooter" treatment – again, I dodged that bullet. There are other, even less likely, types of catheter-related urethral narrowings that can happen – more about that later.

While you are in the hospital, the friendly nurses and nurses' aides oversee the care and management of your catheter and its attendant urine bag. Unfortunately, the catheter is going to be in for a couple of weeks and (fortunately) you are going to be in the hospital only for a day or two. Before you leave the hospital they give you a crash course in catheter management. I'm glad DSW was listening, because only between us did we manage to get the job done that first night at home.

It's all a matter of learning the plumbing. That first night the learning curve was a little high. Not unexpectedly, I was a little woozy and subsequently a little chilled and shaky sitting more or less naked on the toilet trying to get the end of hose "A" into the appropriate end of hose "B" (somehow, at the time, it didn't seem appropriate to use the terms "male" and "female" ends) without dribbling urine all over the bathroom. Undoubtedly there are other similar circumstances that strip a man of his dignity, but that one rated right up there in the "helpless old man" category.

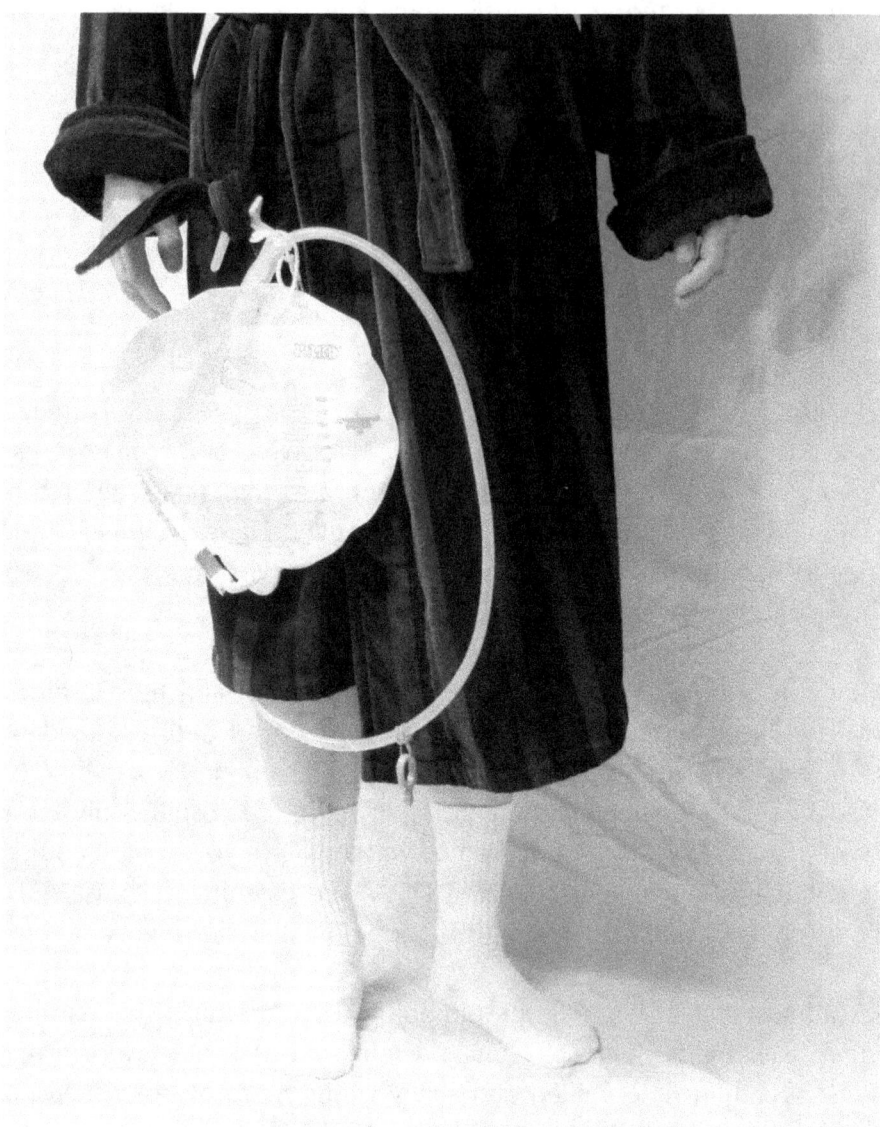

Figure 4 - The around the house urine bag arrangement. In addition to hooking the bag onto the tie of a robe, the bag can be conveniently attached to the edge of a chair or the side of a bed. The object of course is to fasten the bag to something that is lower than the bladder. Try as it might, urine does not flow uphill.

As she would do more than once in this adventure, DSW stepped into the breach and deftly handled the necessary plumbing adjustments.

I had considered sleeping in another bed during the acute convalescence, but DSW insisted that I try sleeping in our bed. Hers was a simple gesture that carried a message of "things are going to get back to normal." It proved to be the right decision, given adequate drugs to ensure both pain control and sleep, and sufficient plumbing to no longer worry about having to get up to pee.

By the next day the catheter routine was beginning to establish itself. The end of the garden hose exiting from my little buddy was affixed to a Velcro band, a little like a garter belt, which encircled either my right or left thigh (alternating back and forth daily). From the "female" end of the catheter tube, the "male" end of the tube from the urine bag was attached.

The urine bags came in two types. The big gallon- sized one was for use during sleep or for walking around the house in a robe or pajamas. (Fig. 4) This large bag has a big plastic hook that could be attached to the side of the bed, handles in the shower, cabinet pulls, robe ties, or just about anything handy that is lower than your bladder – pee does not flow uphill well.

Although this large bag makes for a nifty little accessory, most people find it uncomfortable to watch someone in public casually walking around -- or just sitting there, for that matter -- with a sloshing bag of urine hooked to the pocket of their jeans or attached to the end of a park bench.

For those public outings, the clever pee plumbers have invented the "leg bag." (Fig. 5) The leg bag is about the dimensions of an IV bag at the hospital, and straps to your calf with Velcro straps that are cleverly designed never to exactly match up while you are trying to get the damn thing fastened to your leg.

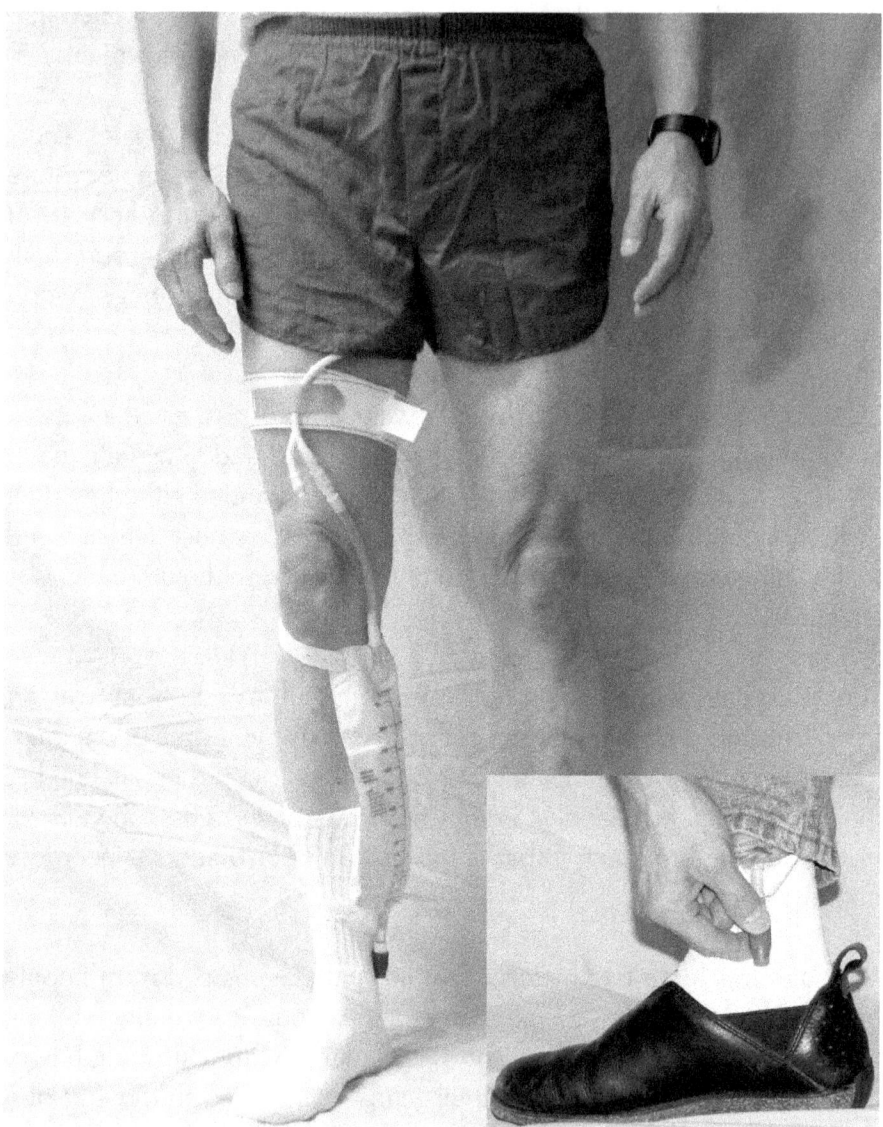

Figure 5 - The leg bag option in operation. One end of the Foley catheter, as seen in Figure 2, is firmly anchored in the bladder, while a band around the thigh secures the open end. If not before, you will be a boxer guy during the catheter phase of your recovery. The bag is hopefully securely strapped to the lower leg. The inset shows a well-turned ankle and the business end of the bag. It should be obvious that inattention to detail while emptying the bag will result in a yellow sock and a shoe full of urine.

Unless you are wearing tight pants -- and believe me, no one with a catheter would ever want to wear tight pants -- the tubing and leg bag are largely invisible to anyone but that Sherlock Holmes type who notices one pant leg ruffles more when you walk than the other.

I mentioned earlier the problems with the leg bag straps; this is more than just an idle concern. You most likely will lose significant points in a social setting when a bag of urine suddenly falls out of your pants, particularly while you are walking. With sufficient slack in the tubing, all you need suffer is a little social embarrassment. If, however, the bag drops far enough south to put stress on the tube "A" to tube "B" junction, other problems may arise. If you had pushed the two ends together sufficiently firmly, you will become acutely aware of that little water- filled balloon trying to exit your body, not tight enough with the junction -- and now you have a blossom of wetness starting on your thigh and spreading down your leg. Bottom line – get the straps on the bag fastened tightly.

Despite its potential problems, the leg bag is the catheter-wearer's ticket out of the house and back into the real world. Ten days after my surgery the leg bag let me travel several hours in a car and then testify in court for a few hours with no worries about bathroom breaks.

Which isn't to say that there aren't number-1 type bathroom breaks. The bags do get full and the conventional wisdom is that the bags shouldn't be allowed to get too full or left unemptied for too long. The big worry is that bacteria will get settled either in the bags or tubing, and climb back up into the bladder to cause all sorts of havoc. To prevent this there is a daily routine of flushing the bags and tubing with soapy water and occasionally with vinegar. They give you a nifty big syringe to do this with - which can subsequently be used quite effectively in water fights.

No one told me, most likely because it doesn't exist, what the proper etiquette is for emptying a urine bag in a public toilet. Since you don't go out with the large bag, this applies primarily to the leg bag. The actual emptying is relatively easy. At the bottom of the bag is a stop-cock (how appropriate) that you simply open and whoosh, your bag is empty. You will only once forget that the end of the emptying tube and your shoe are right next to each other (see Fig. 5 again).

I felt it was best to empty the bag into the toilet while using a public (or private) restroom. However, occasionally the toilet stalls were all occupied. I sometimes suffer from "shy bladder" syndrome, but it never did bother me to sidle on up to a urinal, lift my foot up to the edge, and flip the switch. It was amazing to watch the guys next to you trying hard not to watch. I suspect that Fido would have been proud of my lifting technique, but he never would have quite understood why the pee was coming out of my leg.

So far, I have made it sound like the catheter wasn't much more than a nuisance, and for some, that's true. My catheter and I, however, hated each other. The rub's the rub. Basically, the external tubing part of the process was really nothing more than a nuisance. All but a couple inches of the internal part of the tubing was innocuous. But the interface between the tubing and the end of me was a war zone.

The trick was to achieve a perfect synch between the catheter and my little buddy. When they became out of synch, then the tube and the last few inches of little buddy rubbed against each other. I don't think the tube cared, but little buddy most certainly did.

It started out as a minor discomfort, but as the days went by and the same few inches of my poor abused little buddy kept getting abraded by the garden-hosed yellow rubber monster, "discomfort" passed into the new zone of "this fucking hurts like hell."

The solution was to achieve perfect harmony between catheter and penis. That was possible, but it in essence required me to be largely immobile. With proper adjustment, it could be done at night in bed, sitting in a chair (which was always preceded by a moment of intense dysynchrony as you sat down), and standing upright but stationary.

Moving from point "A" to point "B" was a challenge. It was "possible" to walk briskly and perhaps even run a little, but it took only a few seconds of wondering why your penis was on fire to realize those were activities to avoid (plus there was a very real risk that your leg bag would fly off).

What developed was the "catheter shuffle." Jack had a very useful handout for the post-prostatectomy patient (see the Appendix). He recommended wearing bib overalls for the first several days. It was an excellent suggestion. Loose baggy clothes minimized the effect of the pants themselves pushing the catheter tube out of synch. Since bending the leg at the groin inherently moved the catheter against little buddy, the next requisite was to walk stiff-legged. I don't know how many *Gunsmoke* fans are still left out there, but I did a good Festus imitation for the duration of those two weeks.

From the stares, I know that I cut quite a figure as I slowly shuffled down the corridors of the hospital in my Dickey's bib overalls with my physician's badge dangling incongruously around the collar of my flannel shirt. And if there were stares in the hallways, there were outright gawks in the physicians' lounge. The amazing thing was that no one asked why I was shuffling around in bib overalls. In response to one persistent silent gawker, I hoisted up a pant leg on the urine bag side and was rewarded with an quizzical gawk transformed into a very impressive open-mouthed "Oh!"

One of the seminal (I know it's a bad pun – the seminal glands that provide some of the seminal fluid are also removed with the prostate) moments in a post-prostatectomy patient's recovery is the moment the catheter comes out. It was like a birthday and Christmas all wrapped up into one when my two-week anniversary arrived (actually, in a cruel twist of fate, due to the weekend I had to wait an extra two days).

Once again it amazed me how many attractive young women there were working as nurses and physicians' assistants in a urology office. But as far as getting that catheter out, it didn't make the slightest difference. If they had pulled that sucker out in the waiting room, or outside on the street corner, I wouldn't have cared. I just wanted that infernal "thing" out of me. And just like that, it was.

Now that the catheter was gone, however, I once again had to assume responsibility for my own peeing. Here I faced the first of the "Big Two" complications of a prostatectomy: incontinence. Most men don't have a major problem; a few will suffer from chronic dribbling for a few weeks or months, and a very few will have long-term leaking that requires some additional surgery to repair. Yet most men will find that they aren't quite as dry as they were before the surgery.

Should you find yourself talking to a man in the postoperative prostatectomy catheter stage of his recovery, you may note that from time to time his eyes might glaze and unfocus, he stops talking, and appears to be holding his breath. It looks very much like he is going to the bathroom in his pants. What's really happening is that he is doing his Kegel exercises.

Women have been using these exercises for years to strengthen the muscles on the floor of the pelvis that help keep your bladder sphincter closed. Men have the same muscles, but unlike our female friends, a firm prostate and a long urethra buttress them. Take the prostate out, and those muscles now have to work harder to keep a man dry.

Like the ninety-pound weakling on the beach, the way out of this mess is to build bigger muscles, and that takes exercise. So, faced with the challenge that, "If you do this you are less likely to leak when the catheter comes out," we exercise. It's a simple exercise, really; just imagine that you are peeing and then tighten the muscles that would make you stop, like when you suddenly realize you no longer are peeing into, but rather just close to, the toilet bowl. There is some schedule for how often you are to do this, but what it breaks down to is, do your exercises whenever you remember to, and try to remember to frequently. I found the middle of a boring conversation was a perfect time.

I asked a good friend who had preceded me down the prostatectomy trail about incontinence. With a smile he said that things were pretty good except for one instance. "Yah know, Brad, when you're in public and trying to quietly squeeze a fart out without being heard, that's when it gets yah." He's right.

Although well aware of the possibility of some incontinence, at the moment the catheter comes out, you feel like a player on some "Spin the Dribbler" contest. While Jack's handout did a reasonably good job discussing postoperative problems, it didn't adequately address "What do I do now that I'm standing here naked in your exam room with a catheter that used to be in me now lying in the trash?"

In preparation for the de-catheterizing moment, I had explored a heretofore uncharted area of the supermarket – the "Incontinence Aids" aisle. I had no idea of the array of products. Eventually I chose some brief-style adult male incontinence undergarment – they fortunately are still sitting unopened in my closet.

I definitely recommend that anyone about to under go a prostatectomy seek out others who have gone before him. One such recent graduate of the "Who needs a prostate?" school suggested I bring some newborn diapers with me to the catheter removal. With just a little trimming, the newborn diaper wraps neatly around your little buddy and can easily absorb a little dribbling (for those of you that are boxer wearers – which I definitely recommend during the catheter time – the diapers will require briefs). I suspect more would be needed for a more constant dribbling. The newborn diaper proved easy to carry around in a pocket and was comfortable to wear. It wasn't obvious that you were wearing a diaper, yet the diaper produced a very plausible, and perhaps enviable, bulge in your pants.

The good news was that continence wasn't a major issue for me. Although I could notice a change from before, I pretty much walked away with full bladder control. I wore the diapers, just in case, for a couple of days and eventually gave them up. I had anticipated having to pee burning gasoline the first few trips to the urinal, but even that didn't happen. Had things not turned out this way, the "LD" in the title might have stood for "Lightly Dribbling."

The noticed change was a greater sense of urgency and a greater need to consciously "hold on" when my bladder was saying, "It's time to go NOW!" Occasionally there still are rare unpleasant leaks immediately after I go to the bathroom. Pretty much I'm about where I thought I would be ten years from now. The good news -- there's always a silver lining-- is that it's easier to initiate urinating, which gets back to the old saying about never getting behind the old man in the men's restroom.

Now to the catheter's revenge. There is no doubt in my mind that when I complained about my catheter, those who had gone before me in this prostatectomy saga, and the staff in Jack's office, all thought that I was a wimp; so I sucked it up, tried Lamaze breathing, and shuffled slowly.

Well, as it turned out, my catheter, or more precisely, my little buddy, was trying to tell me something. All of my discomfort (which in itself is a wimpy word for "pain") was a reflection that the catheter had been slowly eroding away the lining of little buddy's urethra. Once the catheter was gone, the irritated sides of the urethra, in retribution for being mistreated, decided to grow together rather than leaving the opening that nature had intended.

The first sign of trouble dealt with a little piece of anatomy known as the fossa navicularis. This little anatomic gem is a small widening at the end of the penis that essentially focuses the flow of urine into a tight stream. In male dogs it allows them to accurately mark a tree. In humans it allows the adventurous to pee through the hole of a toilet seat in the down position. As a urologist in medical school once so succinctly put it, the fossa navicularis is what keeps you from peeing like a girl.

My fossa navicularis was shot. Another urologic gem from med school also said that a man with a good stream should be able to pee over a three-rail fence (which reflects that I went to medical school when at least someone knew what a three-rail fence was). In any case, I could now not only pee over a three-rail fence I could essentially pee all over the fence at the same time. I was, as the old urologist would have said, peeing like a girl.

It was a sign that something was wrong, and prompted an appointment with Jack, but in the short term it could be handled by getting a little closer than usual to the urinal and abandoning stand-up peeing into a toilet.

Have you ever watched a fire hose after it has been attached to the fire hydrant and the fireman then opens the water valve? The collapsed hose suddenly bulges tight and squirms over the ground as the pressure pushes out the kinks. Although not quite so dramatic, about three or four days after the catheter came out, my little buddy started to think that he was a fire hose.

When I started to urinate I could feel the urethra bulge (and for the women out there, we guys have been holding this thing to pee for a long time and can recognize a never-before-bulging urethra when we feel one), it took a bend to the left, and there was no doubt that the volume of urine coming out was significantly diminished. It was like a nozzle on the end of a cheap garden hose. If I manually did the fossa navicularis's job I could easily clear a five- rail fence.

The narrowing at the end of my little buddy wasn't particularly painful – that would come later – but I was worried that undue pressure was being put on the suture line that Jack had so carefully used to sew the two ends of urethra together where my prostate once had been. Leaking along that suture line will result in a little puddle of urine where it isn't supposed to be – a urinoma. This isn't a medical emergency if caught in time, but it is quite literally a pain in the ass. Thus, I was anxious for Jack to resolve the problem.

Upon presenting at Jack's office, when I told the staff that I had a stenosis, they made the logical assumption that I was talking about the more common narrowing that can occur along the suture line. When I initially said the "stenosis" word, they nodded in understanding and explained that the good news was that a stenosis might explain my good continence control.

I'm not quite sure that any physician's office staff quite knows what to do when their patients calmly shake their heads and say, "Nope, that's not what's going on. These are my symptoms and this is where the problem is." They listened politely, agreed that I was probably right, shifted from plan A to plan B, and cheerfully said, in effect, "We have an app for that too."

Jack came in a little later, and as you have to do in any physician's office, we went over everything all over again. Jack then used a small probe to do something that no one should ever do to anyone else's little buddy and said, "Yup, you've got a distal stenosis, all right. I'll dilate it up and give you a needle dilator to keep it open and you'll be on your way." I did not at all like the sound of a "needle" dilator. On her way out the door Jack's nurse, a very friendly and pleasant lady, committed one of the cardinal sins of dealing with patients. She confirmed what I had already figured out, but as she was about to go out the door, why did she have to smile when she offhandedly said, "This is going to hurt!"

I didn't want to look when Jack's nurse came back with her Inquisition tools. First, she shot a glob of Novocaine jelly up my urethra. At least I took her at her word that she did, because if that was "deadened" then I don't want to even think about not having had the Novocaine.

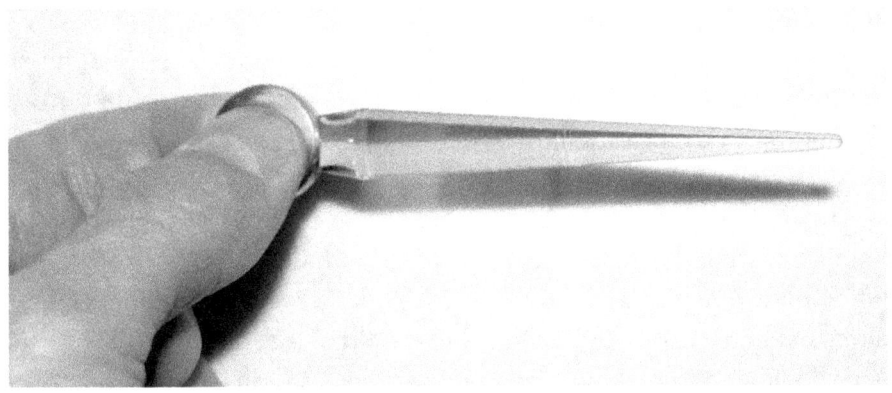

Figure 6 - The needle uretheral dilator. Not illustrated here is the fact that when used on a real uretheral narrowing, the halfway point of the dilator actually enlarges to about the size of a baseball bat.

Jack, with the admonition used by doctors and dentists for years that, "You might feel some discomfort here," then proceeded to insert a graduated series of catheters ranging from regular to fire hose. He then finished up with his "needle dilator." I wish that there was some way to differentiate what exactly was meant by "some discomfort." I mean, that can range from a little gas that might ruin a movie to someone ripping you fingers off. Well, in retrospect it wasn't finger-ripping-off, but it did require some modified Lamaze breathing again, and I was very, very, happy when Jack put his toys back on the table. I do however wish that I hadn't seen the blood on the drape. Little buddies and blood were never meant to be seen in the same field.

The Inquisition, however, wasn't quite over. Jack presented me with my very own personal "needle dilator" to be used in the comfort (?) and privacy of my own home (like, where else would you stick this thing up your little buddy?). Perhaps I should stop here and describe this "needle dilator" (Figure. 6). In reality, it's a rather pretty little thing: a cone of clear blue plastic that ranges from Carolina blue at the tip to a deep Duke blue at the end. The working part is three inches long with a Life Saver-shaped tab on the top to hold on to. At the tip the dilator is only a rounded sixteenth of an inch wide, but it expands to a whole half inch at the base (that's the equivalent to about ten little buddy inches, believe me). The dilator is esthetically capable of being worn as personal bling (it could, but it hasn't) and to this day hangs on a metal chain on my dresser mirror as a memento.

My marching orders from Jack's office were that the dilator, with the help from some KY jelly, was to be inserted halfway up the end of my little buddy twice a day for two weeks. With German precision, I etched a mark exactly 1.500000 inches from the tip of the torture device. I was very dedicated to making sure that the stenosis didn't come back – no way I was going through that again if I didn't have to – but on the other hand, if Jack said halfway, then there also was no way I wanted my little dilator "friend" to go a micron further in than necessary.

At the end of the two weeks the narrowing was gone, and I'm happy to report, has stayed gone. Not that the catheter didn't leave a permanent mark; at full pressure I still can cover a toilet seat, but with a little focus, both mental and manual, the problem is manageable. All in all, I managed to avoid the major continence/peeing problems associated with a prostatectomy. Not everyone is so lucky, but most, after a few months, are. That, then, leaves the other major area of complications to discuss.

Stiffening Agents

PERHAPS HERE, NEAR the end, it finally is time to address the 500-pound gorilla in the room – impotence, or to be politically correct – erectile dysfunction.

I don't think I'm alone in saying that the first thought that went through my mind when I tried to put my head around the concept of "me" having prostate cancer was, "Is this the end of my sex life?"

I'll grant you, the preoperative discussion about incontinence was eye-opening, and more than a little scary, but leaking didn't begin to compare with – it's hard (bad pun) to even say the word – impotence.

DSW and I had a long (another bad pun?) discussion with Jack about what our society has so euphemistically coined as ED (erectile dysfunction). I believe that Jack may have painted a little rosier picture for me than he should have, but then again, he was giving his experience, and not national numbers. The fact is however, nationally, the majority of men undergoing a prostatectomy, even a robotic one, will be left with some degree of ED.

Although he acknowledged the risk of ED, Jack looked both DSW and me in the face and said he fully expected us to be having sex together by a year and a half after the surgery. First reaction? "That's great!" Second reaction? "A year and a half? That's a long non-fucking time!" Third reaction? "Yeah, right. I want to believe you, but I don't."

I'm sure Jack read the skepticism in my face, because he went on rapidly to say, "But if things don't turn out right, I can give you something that can give a dead man an erection. You still will be able to have sex." There were multiple implications to that statement. The one I heard was, "No matter what, you can still have sex." The other implication got buried under the first, but I vaguely remember there was something in there about needles.

The whole ED thing lay like a subliminal cloud of anxiety from the moment of diagnosis right up through the not so subliminal anxiety of walking into the OR. Strangely (not so strange, I guess, if you think about it) however, the anxiety of, "What *am* I getting into?" was gone from the moment I awoke from the surgery. In its place would be the anxiety of "What *have* I gotten myself into?" The beauty of that particular concern was the easy rationalization that it was far too early to know the answer.

For the first few weeks, I lived in a very comfortable state of denial. Let Mother Nature knit things back together again. I'll just let things rest, spend the time thinking good thoughts, and in a couple of weeks hopefully I'll be a stand-up guy once again.

In no small measure this cheerful "let's wait and see" denial was fueled by the fact that a garden hose was still stuck up my little buddy. It's amazing how fast that rubber tube can quickly squash any lustful thoughts engendered by an attractive woman on the street. With interest, I read a small segment of Jack', "So you just had a prostatectomy?" pamphlet, on the perils of an erection with a catheter in place. The thought of that sent shivers up my spine; yes indeed, I could imagine that, as the pamphlet said, a catheter-encased erection would truly be "uncomfortable." I certainly didn't want to risk it, but God, please, let it happen to me. It didn't.

It was about two weeks after the catheter had come out that I decided it was about time to see exactly what Jack had left me and what Mother Nature had knitted. This was the beginning of what I continue to refer to as my "Science Fair Project." As I think about my science fair projects from long ago, this was to be far more interesting than any of them had been -- full of more surprises, disappointments, and, let's face it, just more entertaining.

At the time of this writing, DSW and I have been married for nearly forty years. During that time we have grown into a very rewarding and comfortable sex life that is otherwise our business. But the point is, that's not the entirety of my sex life (no, I'm not talking about other women – or men). I'm talking about the "M" word – masturbation.

And I don't believe that it is just me that gets a little squirrelly with the "M" word. I doubt that there is any topic that is so uniformly applied and so uniformly not discussed. I recently was discussing with a prosecutor that some experts do not use the term "Shaken Baby Syndrome" because there are few - to no - cases where a shaking was ever independently witnessed. I pointed out that by the same logic masturbation might also be so rare as to be a nonreportable event. He looked uncomfortably at his colleagues and said he probably would not use that analogy in court - perhaps a wise move.

Anyway, where I'm going with this is that while DSW had a vested interest in my little buddy's progress, I thought it might be wise for me to have some idea of his performance level before involving the DSW. In other words, my inquiring mind wanted to know first.

Although I preferred to use the term, "flying solo," in any event about two weeks after the catheter came out, and not inconsequentially after Mr. Dilator was done with me, little buddy and I sat down to see what we could do.

With the usual props and methods I applied myself to the task at hand, so to speak. I watched with great expectation, and trepidation, as little buddy slowly pulled himself up to perhaps half-mast, and then ground to a halt, refusing to harden any more.

This probably is the point to discuss exactly how much of an erection is enough of an erection? The answer, of course, is what are you planning to do with said erection? As I will allude to in a moment, if you are "flying solo" then "not much" of an erection will probably do. But on the other hand (I'm not sure if this is a pun or not), if you have something in mind with DSW, then you will need a little more in the erection department.

How much more? That's a good question. As you may recall from the definitions at the beginning, potency is described as the ability to engage in successful intercourse; or alternatively, the ability to successfully penetrate a vagina. Those definitions might sound nice in a medical text, but what the hell do they mean?

It's one thing for the little buddy to be God's rod of your universe. It is entirely another thing for the little buddy to be hanging on for dear life. I'll give you that the former is an important component of "successful" intercourse, and that the latter is not truly "successful" no matter where the little buddy might happen to be.

Not surprisingly, I was a little "down," as it were, about getting the flag only halfway up the mast. I saw Jack for a routine follow-up shortly afterward and was heartened that he chose to look at half-mast more in a glass half-full than half-empty mode. As Jack was quick to point out, many men who do recover potency have no mast at all in the beginning.

Jack actually went beyond half-full glasses. He sounded quite encouraged and forecast a working erection in a year and a half. Statistically, I knew that he was being optimistic (not that I didn't want to hear optimistic); the important thing, however, is that he was speaking not from large group statistics, but from his experience. Ultimately your surgeon's experience should trump the national averages. In any event, I was going to do my best to believe him.

At this point I am going to digress a bit to address the question of "How can a floppy little buddy get harder in the future?" The answer is in the recovery potential of nerves.

A nerve cell consists of a cell body and nucleus and a variably long protrusion, or axon, covered with insulating myelin. The axon protrusions may be very short (tiny parts of an inch) or very long (several feet). Outside of the brain and spinal cord, groups of axons and their myelin sheaths are bundled up into cord-like structures we commonly refer to as "nerves."

Within the Central Nervous System (CNS), the brain and spinal cord, if an axon is broken it stays broken. But with "nerves" outside of the CNS (what we call the "peripheral" nervous system) if the axons are broken they "sometimes" can re-grow.

If you crush a peripheral nerve, but leave the tough membrane intact that surrounds the nerve, the broken axons within the nerve may start growing again down their original channels. What is even more amazing is that even if the nerve is completely severed, but the ends are tied back together again, the axons can send little feelers out to find their original channels at the distal broken end of the nerve and start re-growing down the nerve back to where they were supposed to be.

If the nerve isn't intact, or tied back together, the upstream axons send little feelers out, and if they can't find their severed brethren, they quit. This could conjure up the vision of "little feelers" working their way around the injured area until they found something to enervate. And since the rectum is quite close to the prostate (ask the urologist and he will tell you it is very, very, very close) this conjures up the image of someone becoming flatulent every time an attractive woman walks by. Fortunately, it doesn't work that way. Biologically, a given axon somehow "knows" what it is supposed to do. If within a tiny part of an inch these little feelers can't find their missing halves, they quit looking.

The bad news is, as we knew going into the surgery, that no matter how hard he tried, Jack was going to destroy some of little buddy's uplifting nerves. The good news is that some of the nerves Jack just "winged" might re-grow. Back to the bad news, the concept of re-growing requires considerable patience. The axons re-grow only a few thousandths of an inch a day, and there may be even more lag time as they re-establish where their other halves are.

At a few weeks postoperatively therefore, the fact that the little buddy only got halfway up meant that Jack wasn't able to spare enough intact nerves to get the job done. It would be incumbent upon me to patiently wait to see what would re-grow. Jack was betting on re-growing nerves; plus he had another small ace in the hole.

Even after the nerves have done their re-growing thing there is a phenomena of "recruitment" that might make things better. Sometimes a nerve to penis part "A" can "recognize" that adjacent penis part "B" has lost its nerve. In a gesture of brotherly love, the part "A" nerve might send a little branch out to part "B," and voilà, both parts "A" and "B" are now working when only "A" was working before (although "B" usually will never work quite as well as it did when it had its own nerve).

I, however, was not patient enough to simply wait the weeks, to months, maybe even years, to see if and what was going to re-grow and recruit. What to do while the nerves re-grow forms the rest of the chapter. But first, I want to get back to that initial half-masted little buddy.

Although I was more than a little disappointed (but not necessarily surprised), and it was clear that little buddy wasn't yet capable of "successful intercourse," it was no time for quitters. Flying solo is more about just flying rather than about how far you can get the plane off the ground.

It took, and continues to take, a little more stimulation than before (which isn't all bad), but the "big moment" did come (another bad pun). Even though I knew what to expect, after four and half decades or so of doing this it still was something of a shock to see that the ejaculate well was indeed dry. In the tiny bits of silver lining mode, this lack of semen was a neat trick. Other than dooming the human race, I know that this dry orgasm thing would make it a lot easier for guys frantically groping for a handful of tissue, and would be appreciated, I suspect, by most women far beyond DSW. Nevertheless, even shooting blanks has some advantages over pulling the trigger on the revolver and having only a flag shoot out with the word "Bang!" on it.

In contemplation of my surgery I pursued the Internet, looking for what I could expect afterward. There was the usual stuff about erectile dysfunction but almost all of the personal statements and urology clinic propaganda said that I could expect an orgasm as usual. Only later did I find the postings to suggest what I found out for myself: it's not the same.

I don't want to scare anyone here -- it's not the same, but it's almost the same. Part of the orgasmic experience for a guy is the sensation of moving a small dollop of fluid from point A to point B. Although the rhythmic contraction of muscles trying to move that dollop still happens, there is no dollop. The dollop- making machine is gone. I always hate it when attorneys try to pin me down with numbers on things that are hard to quantify – like, "Doctor, just exactly how many minutes did it take the decedent to die?" So how many "points" did the orgasm lose? It's hard to put a number on it, but maybe something in the 10%-20% range. That's spilt milk that isn't coming back, and I'll tell you right now, I am perfectly happy with 80%-90% versus 0%.

But before I address the issue of my failing patience with half-masted "success," I want to digress to a fundamental issue that underpins all of this discussion: "What's the big deal about having an erection?" I realize that for many, men and women both, this might be a "Duh, is this a trick question?" type of query. There are however many men (it would make things a lot simpler if I was one of them) and probably a much larger group of women who could live quite happily without ever having to deal with an erect penis.

And others might argue, "Okay, so you can still have your orgasms and your partner can buy a vibrator, so again, what's the big deal?" For those who don't have a need to answer that question, I respect that (and once again it would make things easier for me). Yet I believe that there still are a lot of couples out there who enjoy the intimacy of sexual "intercourse" beyond its climactic conclusion. As I'll discuss later, a fully erect penis isn't absolutely required for "intimacy," but it helps.

What I have come to understand, however, is that the biggest casualty of erectile dysfunction is self- esteem. For years I had intellectually "known," but not truly understood, the insult to a women who lost a breast to cancer. From the outside I would argue to myself that what a woman truly is has nothing to do with breasts. Were it DSW who lost a breast, I would love her, physically and mentally, just the same.

But that was me looking in from the outside; that wasn't the same as the woman with a lost breast looking out. Now I understand far better, albeit undoubtedly in only some small way, that our internal body image is a crucial part of who we are. The ability to project femininity can be easily hampered when part of what defines feminine is taken away.

For many men, being able to get an erection and have sex is a fundamental part of being male. It's not that I anticipate I would ever actually have sex with the attractive woman I see across the street, but it is a core of my "maleness" that I "could." Take the "could" away, and it gouges a huge hole (for some) in their male self-image.

I realize full well that the bothersome absent "could" is only me looking out. Looking in, I could fully expect others to say, "You can still have an orgasm. You have a supportive partner, so…what's the big deal?"

The point is well taken. Slowly I have been re-evaluating, recentering if you will, my self-image. The "could" perhaps someday will once again become a "can," but in the interim the once "huge hole" in my male image slowly is becoming more of a divot.

Which isn't to say that I have ceased to fantasize about attractive woman on the street or a naked starlet on the screen, but the fantasies now come with a small sigh and other alterations. These are, after all, nothing more than fantasies, which I have the luxury to modify however I deem appropriate.

A leaking male self-image was not conducive to erectile "patience" for sluggard nerve endings to finally complete their growing back and recruiting. However Mother Nature was going to finish up with me, after a few half-masted weeks it was time to look at other options.

Here is where the experimenting part of the Grand Science Fair Project began. Like any good science fair project, it has involved considerable research into therapeutic options, somewhat controlled studies, and evaluation of results. Like many research projects, it has resulted in a few dead ends, some non-reproducible results, and some overly optimistic initial findings. But, unlike science fair projects in my youth, this has been both a lot more fun and a lot more disappointing.

In a culture bombarded with ED advertisements, it is not surprising that the first assault on a listless little buddy would be from an expected source: Viagra, Levitra, and Cialis. Jack seems to believe, again from his experience with people like me, that of those three, Viagra would have the best chance of improving things. As a new user, I found that the problem with Viagra is the need to take it (for best effect) an hour before needing it, on an empty stomach; so much for spontaneity.

On the other hand, if a little bit of scheduling is what it takes to get a working erection, then I can live with that. A side effect of scheduling however is that the "scheduling" has, in large measure, passed out of my control.

In the past I could, or at least I let myself believe I could, nudge DSW into an amorous mood. Now, with the insertions of pharmacologic erectile aids, the dynamic changed. For starters, the ED drugs aren't cheap. My first time at the pharmacist to have a Viagra prescription filled started with the sheepish feeling associated with buying condoms and quickly morphed into a, "Wow, they cost that much!?" moment.

Okay, they don't cost **that** much, but they cost enough that you don't just take one on a whim and a hope that a "nudge" might get you lucky. So, what does that mean? It means that DSW now calls the shots (which I suspect she always did, but it's a little more structured now). We have once again set aside specific days and times for sex. Even then I can't assume anything until that fateful, "Honey, why don't you take your pill?" moment.

The problem with the above ED pill thing, however, was that they didn't work. In retrospect, I have to admit that Jack never actually said what his success rate was with ED drugs was; he just said which he found to work the best. National statistics seem to suggest that 70%-80% of post-prostatectomy men will not see any initial meaningful response to ED drugs.

I realized that unfortunately I had somehow missed that message. It was with considerable disappointment that after a few weeks of trying the only reliable thing that Viagra or Levitra did was give me a headache. Eventually I just let them molder away in my medicine cabinet.

The Viagra failure was a pretty significant set back to my "self-image" preservation program. This is the point where having a true DSW is essential. Being a DSW, she realized how truly fragile the male ego is and launched her own corrective action campaign. I seemed to have forgotten that sexually active teenagers have been engaging in non-sex sexual activity for years. It was fun, it was intimate, and for a period of time it saved the day.

However, after several weeks of half-masted, it was time for plan "B." Prior to my surgery, when I voiced my concerns about the potential "erectile dysfunction" side effects, Jack had confidently said, "In the worst case, I have a plan that can give a dead guy an erection." I didn't feel dead, but I did want a real, full-staffed erection.

Jack was willing, even encouraging, pointing out that his plan "B" most often was just a bridge to normal erectile function. "In many cases," he said, "this has 'cleaned the pipes,' so to speak. Many men, after using this for a few months, no longer need it." I have to admit, I wasn't thinking months, I was more concerned with the here and now.

Just to be clear, we are talking about syringes and needles. The nerves that I have been discussing do their thing by causing a release of chemicals in the penis that specifically dilate blood vessels so that more blood comes in than goes out: in other words, the penis blows up like a balloon, and voilà; an erection. You can short-circuit this process by injecting the appropriate chemicals directly into the penis. If some of you need to put this treatise down for a second in order to deal with your hyperventilating, I understand.

Jack explained the procedure and assured me that by using insulin syringes and tiny little needles it doesn't hurt a bit. I'm sorry, Jack, but I don't think you have tried this yourself. Doesn't hurt much -- well, I might give you that, depending upon your definition of "much."

It was here that Jack addressed my penis with what I have chosen to be his "little buddy" moniker. I have to admit that anyone touching, in a professional manner, my penis has always been an uncomfortable experience. First, it is the ultimate site of "Don't touch me there!" And second, there is always that little worry that, for reasons beyond your control, your "little buddy" might not stay so "little."

For the first time, I didn't have to worry about the latter problem. Holding my little buddy, Jack showed me exactly where to inject, and more importantly, where not to inject. I didn't like the "bury the needle to the hub" part of the instruction, but the good news was that it took only one shot, not one on each side.

I suppose some guys might have had second thoughts at this point. Sometimes, however, if you want something, a little sacrifice is involved; again, I suppose it depends upon your definitions of "little" and "sacrifice." Fortunately I had done my research prior to the office visit and pretty much knew what to expect of Jack's plan "B."

Implementing plan "B" was going to take a little more preparation. Buying condoms and ED drugs from the pharmacy was always a little disconcerting, but going to the pharmacy with your prescription for Trimix #3 was another thing. (By the way Jack, you should at least call it #9 as per the song "Love Potion #9.") The good news was that I didn't have to deal with my usual pharmacy/pharmacist.

As this was a specialty injectable prescription, I needed to go to a compounding pharmacy that specialized in making drugs like this. I fortunately knew no one at the compounding pharmacy, but on reflection, I realized that it didn't make any difference. I forced myself to understand that in this pharmacy I was just one of many men coming here for the same reason. No one batted an eye at either my prescription or me. I might just as well have been coming in for allergy medicine.

The problem is that they don't just keep this stuff on the shelf. They needed a day to "compound" it so I had to come back the next day (Friday). When I picked up my "I can give a dead man an erection" drug package (complete with syringes) the pharmacist came out to tell me how to store the vials (good for a month in the refrigerator, six months frozen, and protect from light) and to answer any other questions. I thanked her (I don't know why everyone I have had to deal with little buddy problems – other than Jack - has been not only a "her, "but invariably a very attractive "her"?) and assured her that Jack had carefully discussed how to use the drug. In fantasy-land I was thinking that perhaps if she was holding little buddy, showing me how to give the shots, I wouldn't need the shots after all – somehow I doubted both the depth of her instructions and their possible results. She did however, and I'm sure completely innocently, wish me a cheery "Have a good weekend!" as I walked out the door. Yes indeed, I was very much looking forward to a very good weekend.

The prospect of plan "B" injected (another bad pun) another dimension into the mix of sexual scheduling. I mean, maybe you might take an ED drug with the hope of getting lucky, but when it comes to sticking needles into my little buddy, that's something I'm not willing to do on a hope and a whim. When other men have questioned me about the viability of the plan "B" option, one of the concerns I have heard is that "It takes all of the spontaneity out of sex." That's not true. What they really are saying is that it takes all of "their" spontaneity out of sex. That's not entirely true either, but damned close.

I subsequently have had another take on that "spontaneity" thing. People have been rendezvousing in hotels at given preset times for affairs since hotels (or other similar private assignation places) were invented. The movies at least have always made that sex look pretty steamy, so I'm not sure exactly how detrimental a lack of spontaneity is.

But there was another scheduling constraint when using plan "B" for the first time. Jack asked, very nicely, that perhaps the first time we used plan "B" could we please do it in the morning? Just like the disclaimers on the ED advertisements, there was a priapism risk with plan "B" of "an erection lasting more than four hours," as they say in the TV ED ads. I gathered that there was a higher risk with plan "B" than with your usual Viagra dosing. In any event, Jack pointed out that he didn't really want to be deflating my little buddy at 3 o'clock in the morning – point taken.

With little regard to "spontaneity," DSW and I decided that we would send plan "B" on its maiden voyage Sunday morning. The day started with me trying desperately to appear that I was nonchalantly reading the paper. Eventually, after having failed three times to make it through the same particularly dense editorial, DSW uttered those magical words, "Honey, why don't you go take your shot and call me."

I will digress again here for a moment. There had prior to Sunday morning been discussion about who exactly was going to inject whom. I can understand completely that many a man might be concerned about arming their significant others with a syringe and needle and asking them to attack their little buddies. From my reading I have discovered that some couples actually have the partner do the injecting as a part of foreplay. I have to admit, it didn't sound too bad to me, but DSW has a major phobia about needles and made it perfectly clear she wanted nothing to do with either injecting or seeing injecting done.

Thus, I gathered my supplies and retreated to the bathroom. To be honest, I would hope that a non-medical person might have gotten a little more instruction than I did. There is a procedure for properly opening a new medication vial and appropriately drawing up a carefully measured dose; 0.33 ml in this case. I guess that having "MD" behind my name, it was assumed that I could do this. Dipping deep into the memory banks I got the job done (forensic pathologists use a lot of needles, but not quite like this). The injection process would have been old hat, obviously, for the insulin-dependent diabetic. My technique was not only hampered by distant procedural memory, but perhaps more so by more than just a little bit of the nervous shakes. Hitting the vial with the needle was just the first of two moving targets I needed to negotiate.

It is one thing to conceptualize, it is entirely another thing to actually see yourself holding a needle and syringe and your little buddy in the same visual field. My original thought was to give myself a quick jab and get it over with. The nervous jitters, however, suggested that it might be equally likely that I would inject my hand rather than the intended target.

Therefore, I was forced to do things the more difficult way – slowly push the needle through the skin and continue advancing until it was buried to the hub. At this point I would like to point out again that Jack had, on more than one occasion, stated that the needle in question was quite tiny and it wouldn't hurt a bit. I somehow don't think that Jack has ever actually tried this at home.

In point of fact, sticking a needle into your little buddy does hurt. Injecting the love potion #9 syringe contents stings as well. At that particular point in time I would have agreed with those (I suspect composed mostly of women) that argue that what I had just done demonstrated once again that men will do incredibly stupid things for sex.

Injection done, I waited expectantly, and I admit more than a little apprehensively, for something to happen. It didn't take long. Little buddy half-masted quickly, paused for a moment, perhaps just to vex me, and then kept on going. I never have had an erection like this. I felt like the Michelin Man, over inflated by about twenty pounds.

I was impressed. DSW was impressed. We had fun. And then it stopped being fun. In that moment of warm, relaxed, post-coital glow, little buddy was still bursting at the seams. I have heard guys joking about the potential of a long-lived erection as a positive thing; perhaps it is, for an extra fifteen or twenty minutes, but beyond that, not so much. Beyond the first half-hour your little buddy begins to hurt.

And of course there are the other practical things about dealing with an extended erection, like exactly what do I do while this thing decides when (hopefully) it is going to deflate. It hurts far too much to try to delicately tuck it away. Wearing a pair of pants in this condition produces a very distinct bulge that reflects exactly what it is. Once DSW had suggested a post-lovemaking walk in the neighborhood, but one look at me and my pants and she decided that wasn't such a good idea after all.

It was nerve-wracking the first time before I realized that it took about two hours for my little buddy to completely deflate. That time was spent most comfortably, but not in comfort, wearing a loose pair of sweat pants, sitting on the sofa, trying to more successfully read the paper that hadn't been very well read earlier. For the next day I was left with a sore little buddy, which I'm sure was his way of reminding me of the horrible thing I had just done to him.

The instructions that come with Love Potion #9 indicate that it should not be used more than once a day. In my opinion, anyone trying for a daily double could only be described, and then generously, as a hard-core masochist. I personally think that several days' rest would be necessary. DSW and I came to an easy consensus that once a week would work just fine, which wasn't to suggest that the other arm of the science fair project wasn't still gauging the status of an un-injected little buddy during the middle of the week.

Although the injectable Love Potion #9 option wasn't perfect, it was such an improvement from before that I viewed it as a major success. For several weeks I administered the injections, trying diligently to remember my weekly left/right rotation schedule between weeks (I'm not sure that this was necessary, but it just seemed prudent to me to not subject just one side of the little buddy to this insult – apparently there is a slight risk of scarring with the injections and I thought this might further reduce that risk).

In the spirit of the science fair project, I very slowly reduced the amount injected each time, in hopes of reducing the erection time without disturbing the quality of the erection itself. I guess that it shouldn't have been a surprise, but inevitably, one week the shot didn't work. Perhaps the surprise was that I had expected (hoped?) that a dose reduction would just leave me with a little less rigid erection instead of a qualitative move from working to decidedly not working. It was a major setback. Mentally I had decided that the shots were a fool-proof backup plan, and having that theory shot full of holes was discouraging.

I know what many of you health care workers are saying to yourselves at this point. "Stop whining. This is the reason that lowly patients aren't supposed to mess around with their prescription dosing." I mentally kicked myself, accepted responsibility for this misfire, and looked forward to the next week. Although not explicitly stated in the owner's manual, I believed, and have subsequently verified, that a repeat shot (or an ED pill boost) in the face of a failed shot is not a good idea. To add insult to injury, even though he didn't levitate, the little buddy still hurt the next day.

It was at this point that the science fair project began to fall on hard (or not so hard) times. When the next week rolled around, I gave the little buddy the full dose shot and watched in horror as he slowly rose to the occasion only to collapse into an unusable heap. The failure of the sure-fire, "Give a dead man an erection," option resulted in major panic on my part.

Trying to keep an objective, "scientific" eye on this major failure in the project, I cast about for possible explanations. The first possibility was that I had exceeded the shelf life of the vial (which indeed I had) and Love Potion #9 had become reduced to Love Potion #3.2 and just wasn't up to the job.

The next week I thawed vial #2 (supposedly good for six months frozen) and nervously tried again. I can tell you I know exactly what the rocket scientists must feel like when they push the launch button and their rocket lifts only a few feet off the launch pad before collapsing into a fireball of wreckage – for the second time in a row. This science fair project was beginning to look like the one on chlorophyll when all of my plants died the day before the science fair.

Something was clearly going very, very wrong. Not willing to believe that little buddy had somehow structurally changed, and not having changed what had been a quite successful injection procedure, I once again cast a jaundiced eye on the vial of Love Potion # whatever.

On closer inspection, the magical vial of recently unfrozen love juice had small white crystals floating in it. I took the vial back to the pharmacy and had a heart-to-heart with (again) another young, attractive, female pharmacist. Although this might have been awkward, the stakes involved mandated throwing any propriety or modesty to the wind.

It appeared that I was the only unsatisfied customer. The question arose: did that mean I was the only one having trouble with Love Potion #9, or were there others not brave enough to come in and discuss the problem with an attractive pharmacist? I would like to believe the latter, but that didn't address my need to get the problem fixed.

Upon inspection of the suspect vial, the pharmacist agreed that, indeed, the small but visible crystals should not be there. Despite the "Gee, we've never seen that before," response from the vial's compounder, she suggested that in the future prior to use I subject the vial to at least five minutes of very vigorous, arm-rattling shaking.

Trying to adopt my most withering glare, I said, "Let me get this straight. In addition to having to draw this up and give myself a shot, I'm supposed to warm up with five minutes of hard vial shaking?" I'm sure, that in some abstract way, the pharmacist knew exactly what was being done with her vials, but at that moment I believe that she was able to see me, and her other users, in a more personal and less abstract manner. I do believe she blushed.

The pharmacist and I agreed that the vigorous shaking route was not practical (although to be honest, if that was the "only" route, I probably by now would be either looking for shirts capable of accommodating considerably larger biceps, or would have found an orthopedic surgeon to repair my failed shoulders).

I suggested that instead of keeping one of the vials frozen, I would be willing to pay a little more (surprisingly, depending on how much you use, Love Potion #9 is relatively inexpensive) in return for using only freshly compounded material every month. As a result I got to know the people in the pharmacy much better. Whenever a new pharmacy tech would meet me at the cash register, one of the "regulars" I usually dealt with would shoo him or her away and clandestinely retrieve my vials from the refrigerator – it was almost like I was buying drugs of the illicit kind.

For a while the science fair was back on track, but only for a while. It seemed that whenever I got past the first week after buying the new vials, they once again failed me. To come up short was bad enough; to fail lift-off after shooting your little buddy was even worse.

Once again I was back talking to my compounding pharmacist. As I pointed out, "The potency problem here is not supposed to be you." She didn't blush this time; we might as well have been talking about vitamins. She promised to recheck her stock compounds while I continued to buy freshly compounded vials.

The problem continued; in fact, it got worse. A failed weekly experiment resulted not only in a sore little buddy, with no short-term redress, but also dwindling hope for a long-term solution. What I was faced with was the prospect of biweekly, or possibly weekly, visits to the pharmacy. The cost (for me, $30 a vial) wasn't trivial, but it wasn't a major deterrent. I was not particularly pleased with the prospect of long-term weekly visits to the pharmacy. I'm not sure that I wanted to deal with the prospect of eventually knowing all of the pharmacy staff on a first-name basis and getting Christmas cards from them just so I could have regular sex with DSW – but on reflection, if necessary, I would have been willing to do that.

The prospect of weekly injections also was beginning to look a little daunting. The price, both in dollars and inconvenience/discomfort, was coverable, but nevertheless, onerous. It also meant that, without considerable trouble, it was hard for DSW and me to take our lovemaking on the road.

Somewhere during all of this failing injection process I had lost sight of Jack's forecast that the shots most likely were to be a bridge to successful erections and not necessarily an end product. Slowly, almost without my noticing, nerves had been growing and neural circuits recruiting. On his own, little buddy was getting bigger.

After my initial failure with the ED pills, I had tossed them into the back of the medicine cabinet. On a whim I took the 10 mg Levitra sample pack out and noticed that it also came in a 20 mg dose. In the true spirit of science projects everywhere I decided to try two of the 10 mg tablets. It worked! Experimenting secretly at first, it was evident that the Levitra resulted in an erection that couldn't rival a full- blown Love Potion #9 variety, but was pretty close to where I had been before all of this cutting and prostate ripping-out business began.

Confident in success I alerted DSW to the new developments. Given the longer lead time for the tablet to take effect, it took a little more "foresight" to "foreplay" for her announcement, "Why don't you take your pill, honey?" I did, and was rather proud of the results, when, as the Cialis advertisements say, "The time was right."

The right time, however, didn't last long. When the time came for not quite so little buddy to do his job, he collapsed like a wounded dirigible. Buoyed by several successful engine tests, it was a heartbreaking moment to see one more rocket crash and burn on lift-off.

While I was dissecting through the wreckage, trying to figure out what had gone wrong, I remembered a small blurb in the "How to live without a prostate" handout Jack had given me after the surgery. There it was in black and white. I was suffering from venous leakage syndrome.

For reasons that still elude me, when I'm upright (standing or on my knees) everything is fine. When I'm not upright, the venous channels that are supposed to be closed to keep the penis pressurized, so to speak, leak. Thus, despite the best efforts of the poor little nerves to sequester blood in the little buddy, if I'm not upright, neither is little buddy. Apparently Love Potion #9 sequestered so much blood that the leak wasn't evident (or at least not when the shots were working at full strength, which might also have explained why they "failed" when the compound was only slightly weakened).

The solution, in colloquial terms, was a cock ring. Basically, what was called for was anything around the base of the penis that would help stem the venous leaking. You can buy low- to high-end cock rings from an amazing variety of adult stores (either online or in person) or you can go a more low-tech route: a rubber band.

Before discussing rubber bands, I want to say a few words about the store-bought cock rings. For one thing, the variety of products is unbelievable. They vary from what appear to be nothing more than plumped- up rubber bands to pneumatic rings with built-in vibrators (which, according to the product descriptions, purportedly is for her).

For "experimental" purposes only I did purchase one of the mid-range cock rings. One of the advantages that some of the store-bought cock rings offer is that they are adjustable. The problem, however, (for me at least) is that they may not be adjustable enough.

I have to admit that the discussion of purchased cock rings is a little out of sequence. I did try the rubber band method described below first (and last) with my "real" cock ring experiment sandwiched in between.

I was anxiously anticipating the arrival of the cock ring package when it appeared about a week after the order (appropriately disguised and unlabeled). Maybe it is the society we live in, but I don't think I could purchase a bottle opener without an accompanying product insert containing detailed instructions on its appropriate use. True to form, the cock ring also arrived with an instruction packet.

Perhaps without an active science fair project underway I might have easily tossed the five-page cock ring instruction booklet, I mean, it's pretty obvious what goes where. But instead I read the thing and discovered one very important tidbit of information that proved quite valuable. The instruction booklet quite clearly indicated that the cock ring (and thus any other replacement type base of penis constrictor) should be put in place "before" you try to hoist your little buddy from his slumber. Carefully controlled experimentation showed that indeed did produce better results.

The purchased cock ring itself however was a bit of a dud. Ultimately the plain old rubber band worked better.

Selecting the proper rubber band, in the true science fair tradition, continues to take a little trial and error. At first, knowing that the produce people at the grocery store might be shocked, I tried the little rubber bands that they use to clump green onions together. My thought was that I didn't want to strangle little buddy. It helped, but more was needed. What worked better was the rubber band that holds together the daily (but not Sunday) paper.

Despite Jack's statement that you didn't need anything too tight, the truth is, you need to titrate some level of "tightness" that is between "so tight that your penis falls off" and "not tight enough."
I have become a connoisseur of rubber bands. Fortunately the secretaries at the office haven't yet stumbled to why I am often furtively fingering my way through their boxes of assorted rubber bands.

At this point I have found a couple of rubber bands that, coupled with a Viagra, have roughly returned me to somewhat of a "stand-up" guy. Rubber bands break, and I am always on the look out for a replacement band, or one that might work better.

Not that the rubber band is a perfect solution. After a while, it does feel increasingly tight and a little uncomfortable. As my search for the perfect rubber band also illustrates, they aren't adjustable. And then there is the problem of getting them off. I have thought about doing a little shaving, because no matter how carefully you might try to unwind the rubber band off of little buddy, you are going to pinch a little skin and painfully pluck a few pubic hairs. It goes without saying (yet the cock ring instruction manual made a point of saying) it is dangerous to leave your little buddy constricted for more than 20-30 minutes. Perhaps this is something not to attempt if you are seriously intoxicated.

I still haven't ruled out one of those high-end store-bought gadgets with the vibrator – just for her, of course.

Armed with high-dose ED drugs and a stout rubber band, it is now possible to meet the potency definition of "successful intercourse." Even with the rubber band, if I stray too far from head above penis I still worry about wilting. In silver lining mode, perhaps that isn't all bad, since it has forced DSW and me to explore a different repertoire of positions.

I am beginning to believe that the light I've been seeing in the tunnel isn't a train but is indeed the light at the end. This is not quite, but almost, where Jack thought I would be at this point. I suspect that there may be some additional improvement, but I have no illusions of fully recovering to where I was before the surgery.

The status of incomplete recovery does make it a little difficult to deal with the well-meaning inquiries I get from friends and acquaintances about my health. During the first couple of weeks after the surgery I interpreted that these questions largely were referring to how my incisions were healing, how the pain was abating, whether I was back to work…that sort of thing. Later I believe that the inquiries were asking about whether I remained cancer-free and was otherwise healthy.

I reflexively answer questions about my post-prostatectomy status by saying everything is fine. I do appreciate that people are concerned enough to ask. I do wish however that I didn't have to bite my tongue to keep from saying, "I feel great, but unfortunately I can't get an adequate erection without serious pharmaceutical help."

Once in a great while a particularly good friend, or blatant bore, has asked the "How are things?" question and I've given them the straight scoop. Invariably my answer produces a look suggesting that the inquisitioner just realized he/she may have just soiled their pants, and there is an attempt at a quick recovery to sports or weather or some other safe topic.

Sometimes I wish people didn't ask. But I'm glad that they care enough to. In any case, experience has taught that the correct answer is "I'm doing great."

Recovering, even partially, from any loss is a great eye-opener. True, you could pine that things aren't as good as they were, but I'm in fact quite pleased that they are as good as they are.

It is amazing that when you go back to the urology office for your one-year -- and I'm sure all subsequent year -- anniversary visits, ED problems are not at the top of your mind. Without a prostate, your PSA value should be undetectable. If it isn't, then that suggests that your cancer has recurred. As your anniversary urology office visit comes nearer, your PSA status begins to gnaw at your consciousness.

You try hard to push the possibility of a recurrence to the back of your mind, but it sticks with you like the bad smells that get into your hair and clothes after a stinky autopsy. I honestly think that I was more nervous about getting my PSA results back at the one-year anniversary than I was my biopsy result that started the whole thing.

The PSA result was negative; I was ecstatic. Ecstatic not only that the cancer hadn't recurred, but perhaps equally that the therapy to stop recurrent cancer wasn't going to undo all of the progress little buddy and I had made.

I probably would have discussed ED problems more thoroughly with Jack had those problems not seemed trivial in the face of a clean cancer slate. Nevertheless I did discuss the status of the science fair project with Jack, who reinforced the rubber band theory and gave me some more ED tablet products samples to try. (A note on ED prescriptions. The suckers are expensive – somewhere in the $15-$20 a tablet range. Try shopping around; some pharmacies offer discounts. They all do if you get enough tablets for an orgy. As a cost cutting aside – talk to your doctor and find out if you can cut a higher strength tablet in half. A 100mg Viagra tablet for example costs considerably less than twice a 50 mg tablet.I would avoid the online discount sites because the quality of the drugs can be a question.)

As I was leaving the exam room, samples in hand, the nurse said, "Wait, let me give you a paper bag for those." It was a nice gesture, but really, just what exactly do you think a guy coming out of a urologist's office has in a paper bag? Nevertheless I thanked her and took advantage of the bag. After all, it could have been one of those penis sucker-up gadgets that I fortunately never had the opportunity to try.

The science fair marches on, hopefully now in the consolidation of data phase. There continues to be slow improvement with occasional setbacks. Slowly I believe that I'm getting to the point one of my post-prostatectomy friends made when I asked him about his surgery: "I feel great -- who needs a prostate, anyway?"

Epilogue

TWO YEARS AND more PSA tests have come and gone, foreshadowed by anxiety, quenched by a negative result. I've made another major discovery: elastic hair ties. They are almost perfect in size and much softer and easier to use than rubber bands. I hate to imagine what my pony-tailed daughter will think of this, should she screw up enough courage to read this far.

Acknowledgments

I would like to acknowledge Dr. Darlys Hofer for his editorial comments and for being a gifted surgeon. And grateful thanks to Teri, who made the pictures possible.

Appendix

(Used with permission of Urology Specialists, Chartered, Sioux Falls, SD)

What to Expect After Your Operation Called Radical Retropubic Prostatectomy

When you return to your room after leaving the postoperative recovery room, a skilled and attentive nursing team dedicated to having you functioning as quickly as possible will care for you. Being alert and able to follow directions and to learn what to expect during convalescence will be a priority. A special program of pain control will be instituted. You should breathe deeply to expand your lungs as much as possible from time to time. Early walking and early resumption of diet will be encouraged. **Foot and leg movement** and **early walking** are encouraged to promote both good blood flow in your legs and especially good return of blood in the veins. A very serious complication is the clotting of blood in a leg vein. Clots may break away and go to the lungs, shutting off blood flow to the lungs. This event is known as a pulmonary embolus and can be life threatening. So, every effort is encouraged to get you moving, walking in the hallways, and out of the hospital as soon as possible. Lying around too long in a hospital bed can be dangerous. Early discharge from the hospital is also encouraged so that you avoid acquiring hospital-based infections, some very threatening and difficult to treat. After surgery, numbness in the legs, arms, or hands is most often related to the period of anesthesia and is self-limited. Nevertheless, you should report any numbness to your nurse or doctor so that it can be followed closely.

You will leave the hospital with your prostate gland removed for localized cancer. At a minimum, the healing period lasts about 2 months following surgery.

As you leave you will have a catheter to be removed about 10-14 days after the surgery. If straining to have a bowel movement makes the urine turn red, do not worry. This should clear without any problem. Just maintain an adequate intake of fluid. As you go out of the hospital, you may possibly have some abdominal swelling and tenderness. A very loose pair of old trousers or sweat pants supported by suspenders wom under your shirt is useful. One of the most comfortable forms of clothing are soft, cotton bib overalls like Dickies. Bib overalls can be worn without underpants. Just have 2 of them so you can change as necessary. A loose fitting shirt or jacket works well to cover all under whatever pants are selected. Loose clothing will keep any pressure off the tender area. Please avoid elastic constriction of the wound from underpants or other garments. Elastic constriction can set up infection in the wound. If there is no choice, then make sure you insert some sterile padding between the wound and the elastic. A large beach towel or pad to cover the car seat for the ride home is a good idea. Some patients develop swelling of the scrotum and penis. The scroturn can become a big, swollen and tense "bag." The skin may turn "black and blue." Don't be worried. Swelling usually subsides in a rnatter of days and skin color will gradually return to nonnal. Always keep the external genitalia out in front of the legs and never let it get stuck behind or between the legs when sleeping. If the swelling is pronounced you may be more cornfortable with brief type shorts rather than boxers. A scrotal supporter can be worn but the elastic band around the waist must be padded where it is applied to the wound. Some people have reported discomfort while sitting and one patient found that an inflatable airline neck pillow to sit on was very effective for the ride home.

Skin Incision-The skin incision is closed with absorbable suture or staples. If there are staples, an appointment will be made to have these removed. Adhesive, non-allergenic paper Steri-Strips may be applied to the skin to provide stability to the skin edges while initial healing is taking place and the skin incision gains strength. You may shower. Just let the Steri-Strips come off on their own. Under the skin incision, especially at the top or bottom, you may feel, during the 6-8 weeks after surgery, a hard bulge that is not painful. This bulge involves swelling in the tissues of the incision through the abdominal wall beneath the skin. The bulge is sometimes called a "healing ridge." In time the swelling will regress and the wound area will flatten out. If you experience other types of swelling, painful redness at the wound edges, clear drainage or pus, please see a physician. This may be cellulitis or wound infection and needs treatment.

Urinary catheter instruction: You will be dismissed from the hospital with a urinary catheter that is called a "Foley catheter." You will be dismissed from the hospital with a urinary catheter that is called a "Foley catheter." The catheter is held in the bladder and does not come out because there is, at the end of the catheter within the bladder, a balloon, which keeps the catheter from falling out. After you leave the hospital, it is very important that no tension be applied to the catheter or the balloon. Undue tension may result in the balloon being forcefully drawn through the bladder neck and into the urethra causing disruption of the suture line that holds the bladder opening to the urethra or tube that goes through the penis. Do not be concerned if urine, or a mixture of urine and bloody discharge, occasionally leaks out around the catheter. This is usually due to bladder spasm, which is to be expected. Just keep things clean with a wash rag. The presence of a Foley catheter and a balloon in the bladder may produce bladder spasms, and these bladder spasms can be annoying. They usually get better with time. Medication to help relieve these spasms can be prescribed if necessary.

During the daytime, you have been instructed to wear a leg bag and a leg strap. The leg bag should be positioned on the leg such that there is slack in the catheter between where it attaches to the leg strap and where it comes out of the penis. The catheter must never be snagged, yanked, or pulled. At nighttime, use the leg strap and a night drainage bag. The leg strap should be applied securely to the drainage tubing very close to the catheter so that during the night if there is any pull on the bag, the leg strap will take the force of the tugging. There should be satisfactory slack in the Foley catheter from the point of attachment to the drainage tubing and the penis. Make sure that your night bag and your leg bag are lower than you bladder because if they are not your bladder may go into spasm, causing the type of leakage that has been described. The leg bag can be positioned with straps above and below the knee, or the leg bag can be worn with both straps below the knee if there is an extension hose. This latter setup is often most convenient for patients about to fly on an airplane; it is very easy to empty the leg bag by pulling up the pant leg. The straps to hold the leg bag should be positioned with just the right amount of tension and never so tight as to leave deep marks in the skin. If the tension is excessive, the flow of blood in the surface veins of the legs could be interfered with, and there could be an increased risk of phlebitis.

From time to time, you may note that the urine becomes blood-tinged. Do not worry about this. Sometimes the bladder will have a quick contraction or spasm and urine and blood may come out around the catheter rather than through it. These occurrences are normal during the time the catheter is in place as long as it is not excessive so do not become unduly alarmed. Excessive activity when the catheter is in place may cause bleeding to the point of formation of clots that will need to be irrigated out if possible.

Sometimes it is necessary to go to the doctor for his help in removal of clot. You should not take aspirin while the catheter is in place. Discharge around the catheter can also be noticed when having a bowel movement or straining. Bowel ease and regularity should be maintained with stool softeners and other means as necessary. If there is no bowel movement within 3 days of discharge, drink a small bottle of citrate of magnesia. This should do the trick. Sometimes excessive activity can cause bleeding from the bladder lining because the tip of the Foley catheter irritates the bladder lining. If you develop bleeding to the point that clots occur, you will need to moderate your activity and be prepared to seek assistance with irrigating the catheter should it become plugged. It is usually possible lbr small clots to pass. Rarely, large clots fbrm, and you may need to have a physician assist you, but this would be extremely rare.

The indwelling Foley catheter bridges the healing valve and if the catheter plugs and can't be irrigated, only a urologist under special circumstances should remove and try to replace the catheter. Untrained personnel should not remove the Foley catheter unless directed by your surgeon. Replacement of the Foley catheter by untrained personnel may result in disruption of the healing anastomosis between bladder and urethra. This could lead to permanent loss of urinary control. If a urologist cannot replace the standard Foley catheter, he will likely be prepared to use a flexible cystoscope and a guidewire to find the correct continuity between the urethra from below and the bladder above. He will then insert a special Foley catheter over the guidewire and you will keep this Foley catheter in place until it is time to remove your catheter. Any instrumentation or the placement of a new catheter should receive appropriate antibiotic coverage.

You may either return to Urology Specialists for catheter removal when the time comes, or this may be performed by your local physician. If you return to Urology Specialists for catheter removal, it is best to return wearing old clothes (sweatpants recommended) so that you don't soil your good clothes. At the time of catheter removal, the bladder has not been filled and has been collapsed for the length of catheterization. At the same time, the outlet has been kept open by the catheter. All of the tissues including the bladder and valve mechanism have lots of swelling and do not have the normal elasticity that can be expected after the healing is completed. At first, you may find yourself leaking and unable to hold any urine whatsoever. All of the urine may leak out. Gradually, as the swelling in the tissues subsides and the normal elasticity, muscle strength, nerve control, and bladder capacity return, urinary control should return progressively. The time for this to occur varies widely from patient to patient. Some patients immediately have no leakage and other patients take quite a number of months. At the beginning, putting Pampers or Huggies or other very absorbent pads inside a Depends brief may be necessary. There is a pad called the Poise pad that has very favorable absorbency characteristics. The number of changes necessary will depend on how wet the pads get. It is desirable to avoid skin irritation or redness like diaper rash. A zinc oxide ointment can be used on the skin if necessary. While an external collecting device could be used, if you can get along without it, that would be best because you may develop urinary control much faster. When patients become dependent on external collecting devices, their muscle tone seems not to return as fast as possible.

Ointment-After surgery while still in the hospital, Bacitracin ointrnent may be applied by a your nurse to the opening at the tip of the penis to reduce irritation from the catheter when you are moving about and to prevent bacterial infection. Usually, the Foley catheter is left indwelling for I 0- 14 days following surgery, and in order to prevent irritation at the tip of the penis where the catheter comes out, it is important to keep the catheter well lubricated with ointrnent. When you leave the hospital you should purchase an ointment called Neosporin or Polysporin over the counter. As long as you have no allergy to one of the Polysporin ingredients (the antibiotics: neomycin,bacitracin, and polymyxin B), apply a small amount twice a day, morning and evening. If, despite applying this ointment you develop a rash, or significant red irritation, you may have developed a fungal infection. If so, you will need to obtain an ointment like Mycolog or Lotrimin to treat the fungal infection. Another reason for rash is skin allergy to one of the Polysporin ingredients. Do not use Vaseline as a lubricant. Once the catheter is out, hot bath soaks should bring soothing relief to subsiding inflammation at the tip of the penis.

Muscle Exercises are Important after Surgery-Please see the muscle exercises described below. Try to do these exercises faithfully and religiously. They are a life-long consideration. When muscles lie dormant, they atrophy or shrink, and by active exercise the strength of these muscles can be reactivated and hopefully increased. This could be very important in your achievement of full urinary control and good bladder floor support. These exercises, like calisthenics, are recommended as a part of life every year after surgery. Above all' do not get discouraged and do not be frightened by loss of urrnary control. Do what you have to do to stay as dry as possible and be patient as you heal. Urinary control usually appears first at night and then progressively becomes better during the day. Urinary control may be better in the morning when the muscles are well rested.

Exercise for the Muscles to Help Prevent Leakage of Urine

The muscles that need exercise after removal of the prostate are located around the anal canal and the back of the penis. Exercise will improve the condition of these muscles by increasing both tone and strength. Aller many years these muscles rnay be weak, and exercise could help.

There are 2 groups of muscles on which to concentrate your exercise. These 2 groups are to be tightened one right after the other.

The first muscle is around the anal canal. This is the muscle you tighten when you suddenly want to stop a bowel movement, or suddenly want to stop the flow of urine.

The second muscle is around the back of the penis. This is the muscle you use to expel the final drops of urine at the end of urination. When you tighten these muscles you may have the sensation that the penis is being pulled closer to the body.

In order to perform the exercise correctly, tighten first the set of muscles around the anal canal, and hold this muscle tight while you tighten the second set of muscles. Try to hold both sets of muscles as tight as possible for a count of 10 seconds.

We suggest you try to do a sequence of 6 exercises in the evening before bed and rest for 1 minute between each exercise.

One convenient way to do the exercise is to sit on the commode (toilet seat) and relax. Tighten the muscles in sequence as described and hold the muscles very tight for the count of " 10." Then relax prior to the next set of exercises.

These exercises can start in the hospital or with the Foley catheter in place. The best time to do the exercise is before bed so that the muscles can then rest during the night. You also will want to hold these muscles tight when rising from a sitting to a standing position during the day, or when you are attempting to lift something.

Once achieving satisfactory urinary control by performing these exercises, it is important to continue to keep the muscles of the pelvic floor in good condition, so from time to time it is good to continue to do the exercises. Every once in awhile a patient finds that if he stops performing the exercises, urinary control is not as good and that by resuming the exercises, urinary control improves. I urge each patient to experiment to find the best program suited to his own individual needs.

Please note below what to do if instead of leakage you develop urinary retention and cannot urinate after the catheter is taken out. Under these circumstances, it is importantto see a urologist. The valve mechanism can be damaged by inappropriate urethral catheterization, so only experienced personnel should be taking care of you under those circumstances.

Difficult Urination – If you develop progressive difficulty urinating and feel as though you cannot empty the bladder as the seeks go by, you may need what is known as urethral dilatation. done by an experienced person, usually with a filiform catheter and a sound that follows the filiform catheter. If this has to be done, a22 French LeFort sound screwed into the end of a filiform catheter is recommended. A urethral anesthetic lubricant is recommended prior to manipulation or doing any work in the urethra. Another method is to use a guidewire and place a Goodwin sound over the guidewire. The maneuvers described stretch the area of scarring and should take care of the situation. If not, more may be necessary. Only in extreme situations does scar tissue build up and have to be removed.

Leg Swelling-If you develop leg swelling, you may have a collection of lymph fluid that is medically called a lymphocele. It doesn't happen very often but if leg swelling of any type occurs please go to an emergency room to have the reason for the leg swelling sorted out. Sometimes the leg swelling is due to a clot in a leg vein. You may need to have an ultrasound study of the leg veins to sort out the reason for the leg swelling.

Note: If at anytime during the convalescence at home, you note leg pain, swelling, redness or tenderness, this may be the first sign of a blood clot in a leg vein, or inflammation of veins called phlebitis. If you develop sudden illness with unexplained fever, rapid heart beat at rest, difficulty breathing, chest pain with inspiration, you may be showing signs of rare pulmonary embolus. If such symptoms occur and you don't feel right, visit an Emergency Room immediately for evaluation and possible treatment. Don't delay the evaluation by trying to call your physician.

Sexual function: Sexual function is a very sensitive subject. Operations on the prostate often produce changes in sexual function. This includes operations both for benign and malignant disease. The degree of recovery of erectile function after radical prostatectomy is quite variable in terms of time interval to satisfactory erection after operation. There are basically 2 types of operations for cancer: 1) nerve sparing for appropriate candidates, 2) non-nerve sparing for patients with more advanced local cancer such that preservation of the nerve bundles would expose the patient to incomplete removal of the cancer. In this latter situation, it is correct and appropriate to make sure that the boundaries of prostate removal are wide enough to encompass all of the cancer because the nerye bundles for erection cover the surface of the prostate. Of all cancers of the prostate, approximately 90 % begin in the back of the prostate, and some are very close to the nerve tissue. Prostates have to be removed with and adequate margin of resection so that all the cancer can be excised. When wide resection is necessary, return of erectile function is not anticipated (other rleans rnay be necessary to achieve adequate erectile function).

For patients who are appropriate candidates for preservation of the nerve bundles, time to erectile recovery can be very short and, in some cases, very long. There are great individual differences in the age range of patients who undergo prostate removal. For some patients, recovery of erectile function is exceedingly important and, for others, the social situation is such that there is absolutely no interest at all. Most people fall somewhere in between. Patients who have the toughest time are those who are exceptionally interested in recovery of erectile function but the degree of cancer growth is so great that nerve bundle preservation is not appropriate. There are a number of methods to bring back erectile function in those who are motivated to do so whether or not the nerve bundles have been preserved or sacrificed in the interest of obtaining negative margins of resection.

If oral medications (Viagra, Cialis, Levitra) can't be taken or don't work, we encourage the use of medications called vasoactive agents. These are medicines that make the blood vessels in the penis dilate so that blood can flow in and produce an erection. They help to provide good oxygenation of the tissues. The method typically used consists of an injectable medication, sometimes a mixture of agents. **For those patients who have had a nerve-sparing operation but at 3 months after surgery do not have satisfactory erections, it is appropriate to think about use of one of these medications or treatment to induce erection. Promoting blood flow to the penis is important for anyone interested in recovery of erectile function: this involves maintaining and promoting healthy smooth muscle in the penis and release of nitric oxide to promote**

blood flow and proper oxygenation of the tissues involved. These medications have to be self-administered, and it is very important to have an instructional program in order to do it correctly. Some patients will obtain erections after surgery and never need the medications. The medication is for those patients who have a delayed recovery and for those who have not had the formal nerve-sparing operation. Recovery of erection may occur faster if patients use the medications than if they simply wait for the erection to return spontaneously. Promoting good blood flow by use of the medication helps to keep the tissues of the penis healthy so use of these medications is encouraged but only with proper instruction. The ability to have an orgasm is not normally affected. At the time of orgasm, there is no ejaculation of semen because the seminal vesicles have been removed with the prostate, and the ducts that conduct sperm from the testes have been interrupted. Some slight secretion may be noted from time to time. This secretion comes from glands lining the urethra. Some patients never lose the ability to have an erection despite the surgery. They even experience erection with the catheter in place. Erections with the catheter in place can be quite painful but need to be tolerated until the catheter can be removed. A little lubricating jelly placed at the tip of the penis will help decrease discomfort for those who have an erection with the catheter in place.

Oral medications (Viagra, Cialis, Levitra) have been very successful to-date for patients who have had their nerve bundles preserved but erectile function is not yet adequate. These medications promote an important enzyme system that is important in erectile function. There is a case for taking Viagra, Levitra or Cialis on a regular basis just to promote the enzyme system and your surgeon will prescribe these for you if he feels you would benefit from them. Headache is typically the most common side effect. Do not take these medications if you are on any type of nitrate medication, for example, nitroglycerin. If you have angina or known heart disease, you should not take them. If you are taking medicines like Cardura, Hyrin or other medications known as alpha blockers, you should not take Viagra. Be careful how vigorous you are with respect to intercourse. Try not to allow your heart to race or beat too fast so that you enter what is known as severe exercise. Enjoy yourself but exercise in moderation. If you have any doubts about the status of your heart and its ability to withstand exercise-related stress, please see your doctor for a complete cardiovascular evaluation before taking Viagra. If you are on blood pressure medicines that relax smooth muscle in the walls of arteries, ask you doctor who manages your blood pressure if he thinks it is safe for you to take Viagra.

Once you start taking these medications with the intent of obtaining a usable erection, take them on an empty stomach. Take them when you are well rested, for example in the early morning after at least 6 hours of sleep. Onset of action is 30-60 minutes and you will need to stimulate activity. It may help to stand or kneel at first and plenty of K-Y Jelly will help. Don't expect to get a spontaneous erection. If you ever find that the only way to get an erection is to stand or to kneel, you may have developed a venous leak (blood flows out faster than it flows in). There is commercially available a soft ring that can be purchased to impede the flow of blood out through the penile veins. It is suggested you use the medication twice weekly initially, and while it may work best in the morning before breakfast, don't hesitate to experiment at other times of the day. Be careful not to bend the penis sharply in rnidshaft; use plenty of lubricant and keep it straight. Sharply bending the penis in mid-shaft may injure the wall coverings of the shaft leading to formation of a scar of fibrosis, a condition called Peyronie's Disease. If a scar develops, the penis may have an abnormal bend when erect. Patients who do not have a full erection may be ffrore prone to penile injury if they are not careful.

As stated above, another road to recovery of erectile function may involve the use of a very tiny needle and diabetic syringe to inject a little medication into the side of the penis to stimulate blood flow and erection in those people who need it. With nerve bundles intact, it takes very little to do the job. At Urology Specialists, we prescribe a combination of 3 agents (papaverine, phentolamine, and prostaglandin E-1), and 4 possible dose levels of increasing strength. Using the correct level of medication is a matter of trial and error. The training program, which only takes a few minutes, is very helpful and reassuring so that you do things just right. An overdose can cause persistent erection (lasting longer than 4 hours), a condition known as priapism. Priapism is an emergency situation for which you need to see a doctor right away.

Another method to achieve erection involves the use of a vacuum device for which there are several competing models. This device is often used with a properly designed penile constriction ring at the base of the penis. A video demonstration is available. We have a company representative who is willing to visit with you to provide instruction.

It needs to be emphasized that there is great variability from patient to patient and it may take a combination of steps to achieve erection.

Numbness in the skin of arms and legs-It is not unusual for some patients after surgery to experience numbness in the fingers, hands and legs. During surgery, patients are very carefully positioned and padded to prevent any undue strain while they are asleep. Numbness usually resolves well within the 2-month healing period. Try not to excessively bend the elbows and stretch the ulnar nerve, which typically produces numbness in the little finger and ring finger. Numbness in the thumb and other fingers is related to the median nerve and could be related to bending the wrist. Temporary thigh numbness on the front of the thighs could be related to abdominal muscles pressing on the lateral femoral cutaneous nerve from retraction necessary to expose the area of operation so that the surgery can be done properly. This thigh numbness should be self-limited once the muscle returns to its normal position. If any numbness does not seem to resolve satislactorily, please alert your doctor. It may be necessary to have a neurologist pass judgment.

The Trip Home

1. Whether you travel home by car or airplane, at least every hour you should stretch your legs and walk 1) to promote blood flow in your legs and 2) to prevent pooling of blood that could lead

to clot formation in the leg veins followed by clots going to the lungs from the legs (pulmonary emboli). Pulmonary emboli can be life threatening. Elevate your legs as much as possible. Suggested exercises:

a. Keep heels on floor and raise toes up and down.
b. Keep toes on floor and raise heels up and down.
c. Stand and raise knees to waist level one at a time.
d. Stand and raise yourself up and down on your toes.

2. Wear the support hose (white leg stockings).

3. Stay well hydrated during your journey especially in hot weather. Urine should be only the very palest yellow to essentially clear in color.

Exercise restrictions- As you leave the hospital, remember that it takes several months to heal and that includes you incision. You can do all of the walking and stair climbing that you want, but please do not do any heavy lifting or straining for at least 6 weeks after surgery.

Skin rashes occur from time to time in people with and without known allergies. They can be associated particularly with antibiotics or antibacterials. Sulfa drugs like Bactrim or Septra may be the problem. If you get a rash stop your antibiotic and call a physician. He may be able to prescribe an antihistamine to help alleviate the rash symptoms. Rashes in the groin may be fungal and generally respond to Lotrimin or Mycolog creams. Sulfa compounds are also a cause of unexplained nausea, upset stomach and loss of appetite.

Reminders after you Go Home

1. Drink plenty of liquids. Your urine should be very light yellow to clear in color. If it is occasionally pink, don't worry; just drink more liquid.

2. You need to walk every day, but if at anytime you feel your heart racing or pounding hard in your chest, rest immediately. Take it easier on your next walk. Movement is encouraged to prevent the development of clots in your leg veins, which could become life-threatening pulmonary emboli. A short hospital stay and active behavior at home is important. In so far as possible, "don't sit around."

3. Avoid red meat and pork for one month; these meats tend to be constipating. It is important not to have any enemas or rectal examinations for two months. If you have not had a bowel movement in the first 2 or 3 days afler leaving the hospital, try taking 4 ounces of milk of magnesia by mouth before you go to bed. If this doesn't work by the next morning, take one bottle of Magnesium Citrate by mouth at lunch time. If this does not produce results, you could try repeating the sequence of first milk of magnesia and then Magnesium Citrate the following day.

4. If there are skin staples, they should be removed when your surgeon recommends; usually around 10 days after surgery. The foley catheter will also be removed 10-14 days after the operation.

5. You may shower.

After surgery, if you are placed on some form of hormonal therapy (some patients are; some patients aren't), you may have hot flashes or episodes of sweating that are very similar to what women go through at menopause. Please do not be alarmed by these hot flashes as they are usually temporary. If they are very severe, there is medication that can be prescribed (Megac 20 mg by mouth twice a day) but generally it is better not to take anything. Hot flashes as a result of hormonal therapy gradually go away. It can take a number of months even after you stop hormonal treatment. Return of sexual function takes time after radical prostatectomy. No surgeon can guarantee its return. If you have been on hormonal therapy after your operation, the treatment will suppress sexual function. If sexual function does not gradually return in a satisfactory way within three months of stopping hormonal therapy, you can try the steps outlined above in the handout to recover this function.

Care doesn't end because you leave Sioux Falls. Frequent PSA checks are recommended after surgery. The interval will be determined by your surgeon. In the majority of cases, your PSA should remain "undetectable" (<0.008 if drawn at Urology Specialists). If at some point the PSA rises sequentially, for example 0.2, 0.3,0.4,0.5, then you may have a recurrence of cancer and your urologist will discuss this with you. Three-dimensional conformal radiotherapy may then be very useful in eradicating any recurrent local cancer. There are some cases when the PSA will progressively rise to 0.3 and even 0.4 but then settle back at 0.3 or 0.2 and remain at that very low level for many years. We believe that, in these cases, the very minimal rise in PSA that then stays stable for many years does not represent recurrence of prostate cancer, but is due to some benign source such as periurethral glands or possibly a small island of benign prostate tissue that was left behind near the edge where the prostate was removed. Obviously, your surgeon will discuss the implications of any rise in your PSA with you.

We hope this handout will act as a useful source for you during your recovery. Please feel free to contact your surgeon if there are questions of concerns beyond the scope of this information.

www.ingramcontent.com/pod-product-compliance
Lightning Source LLC
Chambersburg PA
CBHW060634290526
45793CB00001B/250